THE LIFE OF
HAMILTON BAILEY

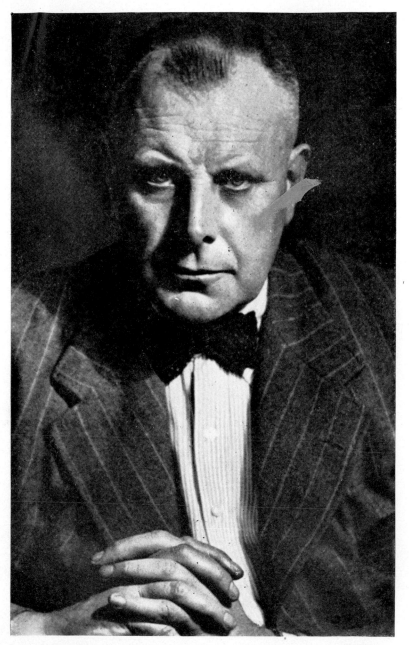

1. Hamilton Bailey, 1894–1961.

THE LIFE OF
HAMILTON
BAILEY

Surgeon, author and teacher of surgery

S. V. HUMPHRIES
F.R.C.S.Eng., F.I.C.S.

RAVENSWOOD PUBLICATIONS
Beckenham · Kent · England

Published by
RAVENSWOOD PUBLICATIONS LTD
P.O. Box No. 24, 205 Croydon Road,
Beckenham, Kent, England

Published 1973

ISBN 0 901812 10 2

Printed in Great Britain by
Grammer & Co. Ltd. Kent Road,
West Wickham

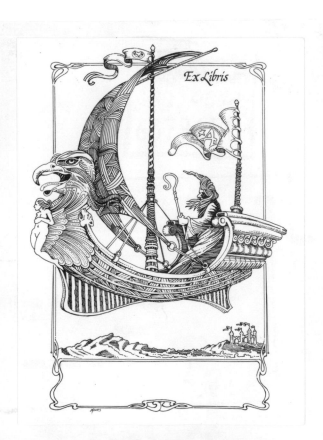

PREFACE

This is the first book to be written about Hamilton Bailey, the well-known surgeon, who is perhaps best remembered for his surgical text books, written with such clarity and illustrated so graphically that they have won world-wide acclaim from surgeons, doctors, medical students and nurses, and have been translated into many languages.

Foremost amongst these is *Emergency Surgery*, which many reviewers have described as the emergency surgeon's 'bible', and which has frequently come to the aid of surgeons in remote parts of the world when confronted with a surgical emergency. *Demonstrations of Physical Signs in Clinical Surgery* is another book which has proved of inestimable diagnostic value to members of the medical profession as well as students.

This biography gives a clear insight not only into the technical skill o f Hamilton Bailey, but also bears witness to the humanity which caused him always to put the welfare of his patients above every other consideration.

His work has been perpetuated by his widow in the formation of a Trust which establishes libraries for medical students in many of the under-developed countries.

This book should prove of interest to many people throughout the world who have reason to be grateful to Hamilton Bailey for his life and valuable work.

Several illustrations are included in this biography which has as its frontispiece a studio portrait of Hamilton Bailey, 1894–1961.

CONTENTS

LIST OF PLATES

FOREWORD

Great surgeons of the past are soon forgotten. The names of some surgeons are known slightly for the instruments which they invented, for the operations which they were the first to perform, or for signs or tests bearing their names.

Hamilton Bailey did a great deal for surgery not only because he wrote 13 books and more than 120 articles in the leading surgical journals of the day, but also because he was a great teacher, and the pioneer of unparalleled illustrations in surgical text books, one of which was written for and enthusiastically studied by isolated surgeons working in far-off places, deprived of modern equipment.

He did not transplant a heart or a kidney, he did not do research on animals, but he devised an operation for removal of the parotid gland as a treatment for tumours which had formerly been considered inoperable, and he was the first to evolve a properly organised method for resuscitation of patients whose hearts stopped beating on the operating table.

His first book, *Demonstrations of Physical Signs in Clinical Surgery*, was outstanding on account of its exceptionally good illustrations, many being photographs taken by Bailey himself. This and another of his works, entitled *Short Practice of Surgery*, which he wrote with Mr R. J. McNeill Love, have probably achieved the biggest circulations of any textbooks on surgery ever written. Over 300,000 of each of these books has been sold in the English language. Both are still being very well revised: the first by Mr Allan Clain; the second by Professor A. J. Harding Rains and the late Mr W. M. Capper. Both have been translated into Spanish, Turkish and Italian. *Physical Signs* has also gone into German (4 editions), Jugoslav, Bulgarian, Greek, Dutch and Chinese.

Yet Bailey, apart from being the name on the cover of 13 text books, is not well known. His life was adventurous and dramatic, with many vicissitudes, triumphs and disappointments which are unknown save to a few of his contemporaries, and even they are aware only of isolated incidents in his career.

ACKNOWLEDGEMENTS

I should like to thank the following for help and information:

Mrs H. N. Allan, American College of Surgeons, Dr Harod Avery, Mrs Margaret Bailey, Mrs Veta Bailey, Dr Marjorie Ball, Mr Francis Bauer F.R.C.S., Mr G. Benfield, Miss G. B. Bevan, Dr J. A. R. Bickford, Dr C. A. Birch, Dr Donald Blatchley, Dr J. L. Blonstein, Mr F. Boothby, *British Journal of Surgery*, British Medical Association, Dr Frank M. Burton, Dr L. S. Carstairs, Dr E. N. Chamberlain, Mr Allan Clain F.R.C.S., Mr L. T. Clifford, Lord Cohen of Birkenhead, Mrs E. Collins, Mr Jock Connon, Mr Robert V. Cooke F.R.C.S., Mr Robert Cox F.R.C.S., Dr Robert M. Croome, Sister June Crutchley, Mr A. and Mrs M. David, Mr J. B. David F.R.C.S., Mr Harold Dodd F.R.C.S., Miss Barbara Donovan, Dr John Elam, Mrs C. Fawcett, Mr F. P. Fitzgerald F.R.C.S., Miss R. Fraser, Mr W. B. Gabriel, Mrs M. Gilbart, Dr Neville Goodman, Miss J. Elise Gordon, Dr Anthony Green, *Guy's Hospital Gazette*, Dr E. J. C. Hamp, Mr Robert Harding.

Dr James Harper, Mr Claude Harris, Mr P. H. Harris, Dr T. E. Hastings, Mr Philip Hawe, the Headmaster of Mill Hill School, Sister W. Hemsley, Sister Margaret Hickie, Mrs Mareuil Humphries, International College of Surgeons, Miss May Johns, Mr R. S. Johnson-Gilbert, Miss B. Jones, Mr Robert Kennon, Miss J. King, Dr W. King, Professor Carl Krebs, *The Lancet*, Sister D. J. Levitt, Miss C. J. Lock, *London Hospital Gazette*.

Mr Charles Macmillan, Dr Pascual Lopez Magana, Mr Cecil P. Malley M.D., Norman M. Matheson M.D., Mr A. M. A. Moore F.R.C.S., Dr J. B. Morrissey, Mr T. A. Nicholson, Mr J. B. Oldham F.R.C.S., Dr G. L. Park, Dr A. S. Pearson. Mr Max Pemberton, Dr Audrey Price, Professor A. J. Harding Rains, Mr Hugh Reid F.R.C.S., Miss Jean Reynolds, Dr D. W. Ryder Richardson, Mrs Ivy C. Romney, Royal Northern Hospital photographer, Sister M. C. Saxton, Mr F. D. Saner F.R.C.S., Mr J. P. Scrivener.

Dr J. H. Sheldon, Dr George A. Shepherd, Mr T. John Shields, Mr E. C. Steeler, Mr Michael Stephen, Dr George W. Stephenson, Mr Lang Stevenson, Mr Valentine Swain F.R.C.S., Mr P. Wade, Miss B. J. Warner, Dr R. Burns Watson, Sister E. E. Weaver, Miss Mary Morison Webster, Professor Charles Wells, Dr D. M. J. Williams, Dr C. M. Bruce Williamson, Mr H. J. Wilson, Mr S. Wood, Dr Andrew Wyatt, and Dr R. A. Zeitlin.

The editors of the journals who have published my articles on Hamilton Bailey with photographs, viz:

South African Medical Journal, Central African Medical Journal, Central African Journal of Medicine, Medical Proceedings, International Surgery, Nursing Mirror and South African Nursing Journal.

1
STRUGGLE FOR SURVIVAL

Bailey's father was a doctor who began as a medical missionary in Turkish Palestine, but he soon returned to England as a family doctor, finally settling in Brighton. His son, Hamilton, was born at Bishopstoke, Hampshire, on 1 October 1894. Dr Bailey was conscientious, liked by his patients, and a keen fisherman, but he took no interest whatsoever in his young son.

Bailey's mother, Margaret, was beautiful, acquisitive, fond of jewellery, and a chronic alcoholic, often picked up in the street and taken home drunk in a cab. She too took no interest in her son or in her daughter, who at the age of 19 developed schizophrenia and was confined to a mental institution for the rest of her life. The outlook for Bailey, therefore, with an indifferent father a drunken mother, and a mentally deranged sister, was not favourable. As a child he was grossly neglected, with no home life.

One of his fellow scholars (now a retired doctor in Co. Donegal, Eire), who remembers Bailey well when they were at St Lawrence College, Ramsgate, tells me that they were both interested in photography (which was uncommon in children of 14 some 60 years ago) and that they exchanged cameras in a schoolboy swap. His early experience in photography was later to be a great advantage in his books. Bailey was not an outstanding pupil, and was inclined to be undisciplined and argumentative. He was not keen on any sport except swimming, at which he excelled. Later in life he played fairly good golf and did some fishing.

When he had completed his schooling, the headmaster told Dr Bailey, who wanted his son to follow in his footsteps and become a doctor, that Hamilton was not clever enough. Dr Bailey, undeterred, sent the boy to a coach to prepare him for the College of Preceptors examination required for entry into a medical college. Bailey failed the examination. When his mother heard the news of his failure she expressed her contempt with the two words, 'you fool'.

It is impossible to know the exact effect of his mother's scorn: but he failed only one more examination, the Primary F.R.C.S., and this he passed at the second attempt. In 1912 he entered the London Hospital Medical College. His father was unaccountably mean over small sums of money, though generous with large sums after Bailey had proved his worth. He allowed his son only £2 a week to pay his expenses in London.

As a student Bailey always worked hard. His notes on biology, dated 1912, are illustrated with excellent diagrams. They resemble the manuscript of a book rather than the notes of an immature student on a strange subject. His notes on physiology, compiled in 1919 for the Primary Fellowship, have about them a professional touch similar to that of his articles and books which started to appear a few years later. These two sets of notes are kept in a small Hamilton Bailey museum at the Royal Northern Hospital in Holloway, London. While at the medical school he won numerous prizes and scholarships.

His hospital studies were interrupted in 1914 by the outbreak of war, when he went to Belgium as a dresser with the British Red Cross. When Germany invaded, most of the Red Cross personnel were taken prisoner. Bailey was sent to work at Schaerbeek Station in Brussels where he dressed the wounds of soldiers (captured at Mons and other battles) who were being evacuated into Germany by train. He stayed at a house where a girl working for the United States Embassy was boarding.

One day, when returning from a shop where he had gone to have his boots repaired, he was arrested by a German detective in the street and ordered to show his papers. He produced his Red Cross card, but this was insufficient, and he was taken to a military court where he was brought before a court-martial. There he was urged to confess that he had come to Belgium on a troopship and was a spy.

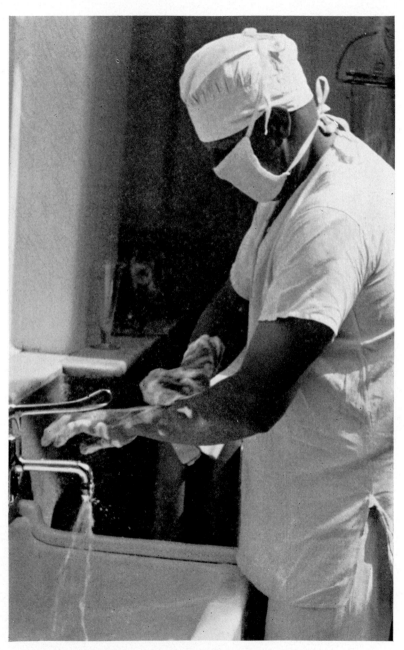

2. Bailey scrubs up before an operation.

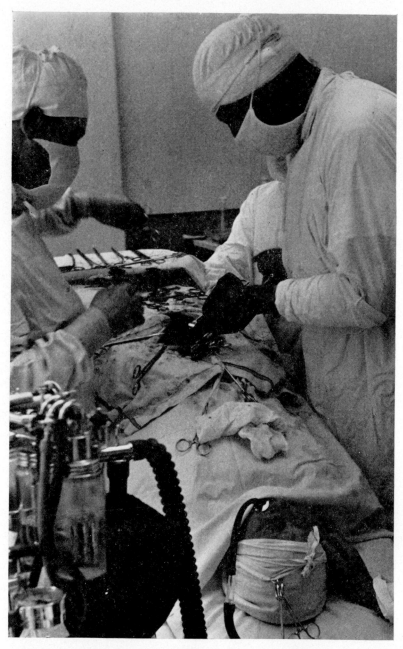

3. Bailey performs an abdominal operation at St Vincent's Clinic in
1946.

Without really understanding what decision had been reached he was marched off to the Ministry of War with other Red Cross dressers, and imprisoned for several days. Two of the men in prison with him were taken out and shot as spies. A guard told Bailey, 'It will be your turn soon.'

Fortunately the girl from the U.S. Embassy who boarded at the same house as Bailey, noticed his absence and reported it to the Ambassador. He discovered that Bailey and other non-combatants were imprisoned awaiting a probable death sentence and made representations through diplomatic channels to obtain his release. Shortly afterwards, the Red Cross dressers were sent back to Schaerbeek to continue their work.

But their troubles were not yet over, for the Germans were extremely suspicious of all captured medical personnel, and all those at Schaerbeek were confined there for 36 hours when it was suspected they were transmitting information to England about the movements of troop trains.

The U.S. Ambassador again intervened, demanding that all British medical students and nurses should be repatriated to Britain under the terms of the Geneva Convention. After further delay the entire Red Cross contingent were herded into fourth-class compartments and taken by train through Schleswig-Holstein to Denmark; from there they were ultimately repatriated. Bailey described his experiences in Belgium in an article published in the *London Hospital Gazette* in December 1914, entitled 'With the British Red Cross in Belgium'. This was, as far as I can discover, his first printed article.

Soon after his return to the London Hospital, Bailey was sitting on top of an open double-decker bus under the railway bridge at Bethnal Green on which was a stationary train filled with Derby recruits (conscripts). The recruits, seeing Bailey in civilian clothes, and impressed by his apparent health and stature (he was 6 ft 4 in), started to shout insults at him, crying out, 'Why aren't you in khaki, slacker?' At once a young woman in the street dashed up the stairs of the bus and delighted his tormentors by delving into her bag from which she produced a white feather which she presented to Bailey. Her action was greeted by the onlookers with shouts of applause.

Soon after resuming his work at the London Hospital, Bailey volunteered for the Navy. He served from 1915 to 1919, first in the Royal Naval Volunteer Reserve until he had qualified as a doctor in 1916, then in the Royal Navy until 1919. He did not enjoy his naval service, and was thankful to obtain his release in 1919 after what had been a boring ordeal.

2

THE SURGEON LOSES
A FINGER

Bailey returned to the London Hospital eager to start work as a surgeon, but there was no vacancy immediately available. He took his Primary Fellowship (for the F.R.C.S.) in September 1919 and was referred. He entered again in May 1920 and was approved. He passed his final in November 1920, and went as a Resident Surgical Officer to the General Hospital, Wolverhampton. A colleague of his writes, 'I can just remember him as a tall, rather striking figure. He did not stay long and I rather believe that he had some sort of a row with the then senior surgeon, Mr E. Deanesly.' Whatever the row was about, Bailey evidently forgave him for it, because Deanesly's photograph appears in the seventh edition of *Emergency Surgery* among his 'masters' to whom he dedicated the book.

Then Bailey became a surgical registrar at the Liverpool Royal Infirmary, where he made a considerable impression as lecturer and coach. His students included several men who afterwards became prominent in their profession. Among them were Mr Charles Wells, Mr J. B. Oldham and Dr Henry Cohen, later to become Lord Cohen of Birkenhead. In the preface of volume 2 of the 18th edition of *Pye's Surgical Handicraft*, Cohen was enthusiastic in his praise of Bailey's energy and his teaching ability both by word of mouth and the written and illustrated page.

Bailey's character and actions were dominated by his tremendous capacity for work, and his interest in it. These accounted for almost everything that he did. When he arrived in Liverpool most people admired and liked him, but they never got to know him. He was so dedicated to surgery that he had no time for anything else. He had no time to make friends and no social life. He thought that cocktail parties and similar functions were a waste of time. He had no small talk and no interest in medical politics or hospital administration. He never wanted to sit on boards or committee meetings.

He was a tremendous reader, mainly of surgical books, and kept detailed notes of his cases – the 'building material', as he called it, for his books and articles. He was sympathetic and kind to his patients in his brisk way, and they had great confidence in him. He was a very shy and sensitive man, with an intense dislike of formality and a positive loathing for money.

Referring to his undergraduate teaching at Liverpool, a former student of Bailey's writes: 'The arrival of Bailey was a godsend and introduced something the like of which we had never seen before. He was a superb teacher of the classical type and we took every advantage of what he could do for us, including coaching classes.

'We found that in addition to his dedication and enthusiasm for teaching he was extremely sensitive, and even emotional and temperamental. Once, on being told that "the portal system is formed by the mesenteric and splenic veins (at which stage he looked cheerful and hopeful) joined by the renal vein" he went quite pale, threw his hands up in the air . . . he ended the class and sent us away, saying that he could not carry on any longer. I have never had any doubt that this was perfectly genuine.'

After completing his registrarship in Liverpool he became a registrar in February 1922 at the London Hospital under Sir Hugh Rigby and Mr Robert Milne until September 1923; then first assistant to Sir Hugh Rigby and Mr Walton from October 1923 to February 1925. He was also clinical assistant to the genito-urinary department from 1923 to 1925. One of his fellow registrars was to become the co-author of two of his books: *Short Practice of Surgery* and *Surgery for Nurses*. This was Mr R. J. McNeill Love. Registrars were generally responsible for emergencies and also did a great deal of teaching. Bailey and Love's excellent teaching made them popular with students.

Bailey's near escape from being shot as a spy in 1914 apparently upset him less than when, in 1924, he pricked his left index finger while operating on a patient with septic peritonitis. The infection was caused by an extremely virulent streptococcus, which killed the patient before threatening to kill Bailey as well. A few hours after the operation his finger began to swell. The oedema extended up his arm.

There was of course no penicillin. The recognised treatment for such conditions was to make incisions in the hope of finding pus. When the incisions were made no pus was found, and Bailey continued in a critical condition, running a high temperature. At last the infection subsided, but it left him with a totally stiff and useless left index finger.

Bailey's chiefs advised him to give up surgery, for they thought that it would be impossible for him to continue. The finger would require amputation; being stiff and immobile it would merely get in the way. Bailey, being sensitive and emotional, became extremely despondent at the prospect of abandoning his one aim in life, but in the end he had to submit to amputation.

During his convalescence Bailey found that the movements of his other fingers, which had also been somewhat stiff, greatly improved, and that he could do everything with his middle finger which he had formerly done with his index. Moreover, his hand was now smaller for the head of the metacarpal bone had also been amputated, and the new index finger (really the middle finger) was longer than the normal one, which was an advantage when performing a rectal or vaginal examination. The smallness of his hand was an asset when performing a laparotomy (exploration of the abdomen), which could be done through a smaller incision. After this he taught that amputation of the metacarpal head with the phalanges of the index finger gave the best results, and used his own hand to illustrate this.

Dr W. writing from New Zealand, described how he, like Bailey, lost an index finger. An infection developed in his right index finger after a surgeon pricked him while assisting at an operation on a patient with septic appendicitis. He became seriously ill and the ruined finger had to be amputated. For a time he was able to continue his work, but later a neuroma arose in the amputation scar.

He left New Zealand in 1934 on study leave in England. While reading *Emergency Surgery* he noticed in an illustration the turned-in index finger of Bailey's glove.

'I recognised also,' writes Dr W., 'that in the amputation the head of the metacarpal was streamlined.' By this he meant that part of the metacarpal bone had been cut away obliquely, so that the edge of the hand came into line with the remaining middle finger. He therefore wrote to Bailey for an appointment.

Dr W. continued, 'I appreciated his kindness and understanding and the care with which he checked and marked the scar area containing the neuroma. I remember his remark "I shall give you a better hand than mine". He arranged for my admission to St David's wing of the Royal Northern Hospital and duly operated. 'The result has been a joy to me, for now I have a painless scar, and a hand which few patients notice is abnormal.'

After Bailey had completed his three years as a first assistant two vacancies occurred on the permanent surgical staff of the London Hospital. For these there were five applicants; Bailey, Love, Cairns, Perry and Huddy. Cairns and Perry were elected for the posts. Bailey and Love, who were two of the best teachers of surgery at the London, were rejected.

3

LIVERPOOL AND VETA

At the age of 31 Bailey was appointed Honorary Assistant Surgeon at the Liverpool Royal Infirmary, and increased his reputation as a teacher. One reason Bailey did not stay long at Liverpool was because, as assistant surgeon, he was allowed only one or two courtesy beds for his patients. He was very short of money, and could not afford a car. During his entire four months as a consultant in Liverpool he got *one* three-guinea consultation. Having no money sense, he rented expensive consulting rooms, and he was still paying off the debt for these rooms for years after he left Liverpool. Had he remained he would probably have become Professor of Surgery within eight to ten years, but he was too impatient to tolerate the position in a teaching hospital where he was at the beck and call of the senior surgeon.

Bailey's chief was Frank Jeans, a jovial man with a robust sense of humour, a gourmet, devoted to the world of the theatre. He was an instinctive diagnostician, and one of the most rapid and spectacular operators of the day.

The Assistant Surgeon's duties were to treat out-patients and deal with emergencies, mostly at night. On operating days he might assist his chief. Bailey's experience was and still is common to many young surgeons trying to obtain experience in operative technique; some established surgeons will not delegate work. The suffering of the starved assistant is a very real thing which must be endured to be realised. When Bailey was accepted at Liverpool, Jeans was on a long holiday and Bailey had a wonderful couple of months. He had about 40 hospital beds for his own use. He was busy and happy. Then the holiday came to an end. Jeans came home. Soon afterwards, Bailey decided to leave.

His time in Liverpool was however not entirely wasted, for he concentrated his energies on the art of diagnosis, and it was there that he did much of the preliminary work on his first book, *Demonstrations of Physical Signs in Clinical Surgery*. During his early days of authorship he kept all the material for his books and articles in large suitcases. He combined his writing with his skill as a photographer, and took many of the photographs himself. When describing any condition he almost always included drawings and photographs.

One of his former students tells me that Bailey was not at that time a very good operating surgeon. Bailey himself says in the preface of one of his books that his experience was still insufficient, and it was largely on this account that he left Liverpool to become once again a resident surgical officer.

During his stay at Liverpool he had the good fortune to meet Veta Gillender, who was to become his wife. Veta gave him enormous assistance in both the production of his books and the preparation of the photographs in them.

Veta is reluctant to describe her first meeting with Bailey. It was in 1925 when she was working at a photographer's studio in Liverpool. She was the daughter of a ship's engineer. Bailey went to the studio to have his photograph taken, and I rather think that he fell heavily in love at the first meeting. Bailey was to discover later that Veta knew a good deal more about photography than he did. They were married on 14 January, 1926. Veta's outstanding attribute was (and still is) her inherent kindness. This was probably of even greater importance throughout Bailey's life than her beauty, or the practical help which she gave him with his work, for Bailey was an enigma whom nobody but Veta could understand. Veta alone could appreciate some of the reasons for his changing moods and discourteous behaviour which he used as an armour to hide the shyness and reserve which so greatly handicapped him.

Veta remained always in the background, never pushing herself forward. When in later years he invited many people to their house – colleagues, nurses, students, publishers, and friends from Britain and overseas – she was the willing and charming hostess.

Bailey was interested in surgery and writing but in hardly anything else. The administration of his professional and literary activities fell upon Veta. It was indeed fortunate that chance brought him a wife so perfectly adapted to this responsibility. Bailey mentions in the preface of the first edition of *Emergency Surgery* that his wife typed every word, kept his case index in order, and helped him to construct many of the composite photographs in the book. Later he was to have three secretaries, dictaphones and tape recorders.

Bailey made repeated references to the help given him by his wife. In the preface of the first edition of *Surgery of Modern Warfare* he wrote: 'The compilation of this book could not have been completed in anything like the time if, as in all my literary labours, my wife had not helped me at every turn.'

4

BIRMINGHAM AND
HIS FIRST BOOKS

By the time he went to Birmingham in July 1925 he had already
had twelve articles published: seven while a registrar at the London Hospital and five from Liverpool. Four of these appeared in
the *British Journal of Surgery* and three in *The Lancet*. His first
article was published in 1923 in the *British Journal of Surgery* on
branchial cysts. The first paragraph of this article strikes the key-
note of his works throughout his life in that it concentrates on the
clinical or practical side rather than the theoretical side of surgery.
'The study of branchial cysts is at once of morphological interest
and surgical importance. In this paper the latter side of the
question alone will be considered.'

And so to Birmingham. He became Senior Surgeon to the very
large Dudley Road hospital which provided him with enormous
experience in emergency surgery. There he performed over 3,500
operations in just over four years, wrote 32 articles, and obtained
publication of his first two books: *Physical Signs* and *Branchial
Cysts and Other Essays*. At the Dudley Road Hospital he had 90
beds of his own and no house surgeon to help him. He was paid
£700 a year with no private practice.

One of his colleagues there, who was also his anaesthetist, de-
scribes Bailey as a 'natural leader whose initiative and original
ideas made him outstanding and who inspired confidence in all
the members of his team'. He was responsible for some important
innovations. He banned the use of talcum powder for the prepar-
tion of rubber gloves, instituted a recovery room for serious
accident cases and for patients requiring resuscitation, was responsible for the routine administration of blood transfusions for
critical cases, and extended the use of intravenous saline.

13

Physical Signs, with 207 pages and 261 illustrations, was an instant success. Bailey himself was more attached to this book than to any of his others. It reached hundreds of thousands of students. But, having read most of his books, I am convinced that it is nowhere near his best, though at the time there was nothing like it.

The illustrations were outstanding as in many of Bailey's books. Indeed, it was he who pioneered the use of illustrations in surgical text books in Britain on an extensive scale, and it was due to Bailey that the quality of illustrations in British text books of surgery have reached a high standard comparable with that in the U.S.A.

The first of Bailey's anaesthetists at Dudley Road Hospital, Birmingham, was Dr Marjorie Ball. Besides being an anaesthetist, she was an accomplished artist. He discovered quite by accident that she could draw, and asked her to make a few sketches. From her place at the head of the operating table she was in a good position to take notes of any points which he wished to emphasise. She continued to draw for him after he moved to London. She remained at Dudley Road until the end of 1962, when she and her husband retired to Pembrokeshire, in Wales.

Bailey first used black and white photographs and drawings, then coloured and very life-like pictures. It has struck me as curious that the illustrations in surgical text books used to be so bad though those in anatomy books were good.

Bailey probably derived some of his inspiration for illustrating his books from the anatomist, William Wright, Professor of Anatomy at the London Hospital Medical College. Wright, like many anatomists, was a wonderful draughtsman who could portray on the blackboard a skeleton, and in coloured chalks add the solid organs, then the intestines, then the muscles of the abdominal wall, finally finishing off with a flourish as he hid them all behind a well defined umbilicus. Of the photographs in the first edition of *Physical Signs*, Veta took more than 100.

I remember how as a student I pored over the pages of this book when working for my finals and how popular it was with other students. It told us what we needed to know more than anything else for our surgical examinations: how to diagnose. Though the book was a success with G.P.s and students, it upset some of the leaders of the profession. They did not like to see a young surgeon of 34 making a name for himself by writing a book which was far more popular than any of the books which they could write themselves.

Physical Signs received a warm welcome from all the reviewers, with one exception, the *London Hospital Gazette* of his old teaching hospital. This review was the first to appear, and Bailey was so upset by it that he did not show it to his wife for a fortnight.

In its criticism it complained that Bailey did not mention Kocher's sign in exophthalmos (protrusion of the eyes such as occurs in exophthalmic goitre or Graves's Disease), an eponym which most doctors would need to look up their medical dictionaries to trace, and concluded with the words, 'This book contains much useful information but it cannot be said to supply a definite want.' Before Bailey left Birmingham in December 1929 *Physical Signs* had gone into its second edition.

He joined the Bruce Wills Memorial Hospital, Bristol, in February 1930 as surgeon, hoping that this might be a stepping stone to a teaching post at the Bristol General Hospital. He was happy at Bruce Wills, a superb homeopathic hospital with good accommodation for private patients. The physicians and staff supported Bailey from the start, and he did well in private practice. But when he applied for the vacancy at the Bristol General Hospital, he was refused.

The successful candidate was Mr S. J. H. Griffiths, who died two or three years later. He was succeeded by Mr Robert V. Cooke, who writes, 'No one could be expected to stay on with that one appointment (i.e. to the Homeopathic Hospital) only. Certainly not someone as promising as Bailey. So it was not a bit surprising that he went elsewhere, despite the fact that he was very happy in that appointment and made many friends who often used to talk about him to me.'

5

ISOLATED SURGEON'S BIBLE

Bailey's third book, *Emergency Surgery*, was published in two volumes. The first appeared in October 1930 while he was still at Bristol; the second in October 1931 during his first year at the Royal Northern Hospital. This is my favourite of all his books, for as an isolated surgeon it has been the most useful to me.

One cannot be quite sure when he first planned to write it, but I think it was probably while he was at Wolverhampton in 1920. He had turned up the preface of his 'surgical bible', *Urgent Surgery*, by Felix Lejars, and read the words of the author, 'I might say that I have lived this book before writing it.'

How much better it would be, thought Bailey, to write such a book, not after having lived it, but while living it. From that day he started to record every operation which he had performed and to annotate relevant cards with suggestions for a book.

While Bailey was a registrar at the London Hospital it was announced that Russell Howard was publishing a book on emergency surgery. Russell Howard was the London Hospital's greatest teacher of surgery, and Bailey probably felt that it would be presumptuous to write a book on the same subject as this great teacher in his own hospital. But Howard, though a wonderful teacher by word of mouth, equalled only at this hospital by A. M. A. (Dinty) Moore, who succeeded him, was not an accomplished writer. His book, entitled *Surgical Emergencies*, which was quite small with only 216 pages, was published in 1924, and went into only one edition. Bailey reviewed the position three years later and proceeded with *Emergency Surgery*, which is today's bible of the emergency surgeon, and is carried on the planes of the Flying Doctor service in Australia and on the ships of the Royal Navy.

Bailey was a pioneer in the field of writing for isolated surgeons. Nobody had done this before to an appreciable extent, though now it has become quite fashionable. Most British surgeons seemed to think that the only doctors and medical students needing instruction in surgery were going to practise in Britain where conditions are entirely different from those in countries where two-thirds of the world's population live: the vast areas of Asia and Africa. The isolated surgeon requires a book to tell him everything which he needs to know about the treatment of emergencies. None can do this, but Bailey's book was perhaps the most successful.

The surgeon at a small hospital in a remote area cannot supply the same treatments as one in a large town. Take for example a case of ruptured ectopic pregnancy, or ruptured spleen, for which little or no blood is available for transfusion. The value of auto-transfusion for these conditions, which Bailey stresses in *Emergency Surgery*, can often be life-saving, yet I have met some doctors who had never heard of it.

In the preface Bailey wrote: 'I have pictured a patient stricken with an acute abdominal emergency and the comparatively isolated surgeon called upon to carry out appropriate treatment. Should these pages help the latter to save the former, the main object will be fulfilled.'

His object was certainly fulfilled when Dr Robert Croome in Canada operated on an Eskimo in the ice-bound Arctic. Bailey learned about it in a letter which came in a parcel with a battered copy of *Emergency Surgery*.

'Dear Sir,' wrote Dr Croome from Brandon, Manitoba, on 19 May 1946, 'I am taking the liberty of sending you one of your books because it has rather an interesting story behind it. You will note its present condition; but that is part of the story!

'I was the medical officer for the moving party of Exercise Musk-Ox which has just concluded its Arctic trek from Churchill, Manitoba to Edmonton, Alberta.

'We (a force of 48) made the trip in 81 days. As medical officer

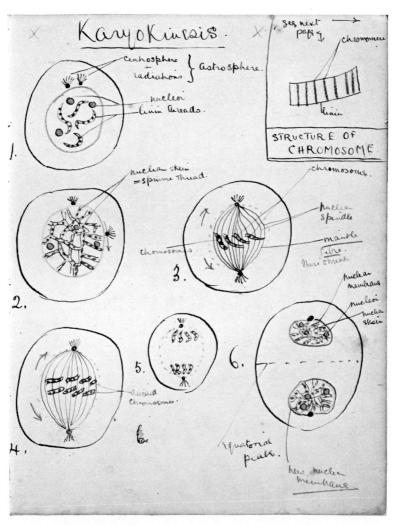

4. A page from one of Bailey's biology notebooks showing karyo-
kinesis and chromosome cell structure. Good illustrations were an
intrinsic part of his books.

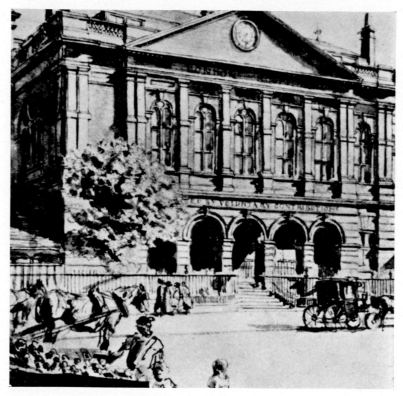

5. The London Hospital in 1917, when Bailey took his final Conjoint examination.

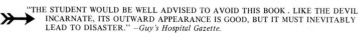

"A really great book." *—London Hospital Gazette.*

"The authors have successfully eliminated all obsolete methods." *—British Journal of Surgery.*

"The Best of the short textbooks on surgery." *—University College Hospital Magazine.*

"Crisp and lucid writing. We strongly recommend this book." *—Indian Medical Gazette.*

"THE STUDENT WOULD BE WELL ADVISED TO AVOID THIS BOOK . LIKE THE DEVIL INCARNATE, ITS OUTWARD APPEARANCE IS GOOD, BUT IT MUST INEVITABLY LEAD TO DISASTER." *—Guy's Hospital Gazette.*

Have YOU seen a copy to judge for yourself?

6. Extract from publicity material for the fourth edition of *A Short Practice of Surgery* by Bailey and McNeill Love (see p. 37).

I had my own Penguin (oversnow vehicle), a medical orderly, a driver, and as a consultant your *"Emergency Surgery"*.

'On 13 March 1946 at Eskimo Settlement, Perry River, I opened the abdomen of a three year old Eskimo boy and reduced an intussusception (in a native's igloo for an operating theatre). I was very thankful that I had your excellent text with me, and very grateful to you for having written it. I have had no special surgical training, and I am not ashamed to say that the successful outcome of the operation was due to your excellently written text rather than to any skill on my part.

'However, the story of the book does not end here. While crossing Great Bear Lake my Penguin went through the ice. It took over 20 hours to get it out of the icy water, during which time the book was completely submerged, which accounts for its present condition.

'I carried the book with me for the remainder of the trek, so that it might complete what we here in Canada feel has been a somewhat historic journey. I feel that you, the author, are entitled to it as a souvenir of the trip, to show your friends where your text has been.'

The copy of the book which he took was the fifth edition, published in 1944. It is kept in a glass case in the Bailey museum at the Royal Northern.

6

ACHIEVEMENTS

Perhaps the most valuable of his many achievements apart from his books was his introduction of a new operation for removing the parotid gland for tumours. For this he was awarded the Hunterian Professorship in 1949. Previous attempts to remove these tumours had been unsuccessful because of the profuse haemorrhage encountered and of the surgeon's fear of damaging the facial nerve. The approach had been made through a comparatively small incision, with which it was impossible to perform a radical operation. Many of the tumours were treated by radiotherapy alone, which was ineffective because most parotid tumours are insensitive to it, and recurrences were frequent.

Bailey, from a detailed study of the anatomy of the parotid, evolved an operation which he performed through an extensive incision after first ligating the external carotid artery. He found that most of the branches of the facial nerve pass between the superficial and deep lobes and could be safely retracted after complete exposure of the isthmus (the narrow part joining the two lobes). Following excision of the superficial lobe, the deep lobe could be removed with little damage to the facial nerve.

In 1970, after his death, Mrs Bailey and I came across the manuscript of a book on the surgery of the parotid gland, together with a wonderful collection of illustrations and photographs. This valuable document would at the time have been of immense help to surgeons, but had unfortunately been overlooked for many years, and has never been published.

Another of Bailey's contributions to surgery was his work on the early and rapid treatment of cardiac arrest. Though this is now a more or less routine procedure in most large hospitals, it was not so in Bailey's day. He was one of the first to recognise the need for an organised drill to prepare us for these emergencies. The surgeon must, he wrote in *Emergency Surgery*, have a preconceived plan of action.

He advised the provision of three sterile packages containing the drugs, the instruments, and the defibrillator, an instrument for delivering an electric shock to the heart when performing unco-ordinated and useless waves of contraction, to make it beat normally. The idea of appointing a timekeeper, a student, junior nurse or porter, to shout out each passing minute from the time when the anaesthetist sounded the warning note of danger was his own.

Another useful innovation was his method of finding out whether the heart had really stopped beating in the absence of such refinements as an attached electrocardiograph. It is of course usually quite ineffective to feel the pulse, for it is all too easy to imagine that the pulse is palpable. It is equally useless to apply the stethoscope to the chest, for imagination here too can play a mis-leading role, and the noise in the instrument room precipitated by the emergency renders auscultation difficult.

If the anaesthetist cannot observe pulsation of the carotid arteries we nowadays apply external cardiac massage (unknown in Bailey's day) while the anaesthetist inflates the lungs.

But Bailey's method for determining whether the heart is beat-ing was the most certain for finding out whether it was necessary to open the chest. This was to insert a long, thin needle, as for lumbar puncture, into the fourth left intercotal space close to the sternum, directing its point backwards into the left ventricle. If the heart is beating oscillations will be transmitted to the needle. If the heart has stopped the penetration of the ventricle may cause the heart to start beating again.

Bailey invented at least 18 surgical instruments. The first, in 1924, was an unbreakable surgical needle. Some of his instruments are still used, and I have myself found them extremely useful.

I met Bailey only once, in 1933, when I went to the Royal Nor-thern to watch him operate, but I corresponded with him several times, and was honoured by his quoting some of my published articles in *Emergency Surgery* and the *Medical Annual*.

Shortly before he died he wrote asking me whether I would like to have some of his instruments. I sent him a short list, and he sent me every one for which I asked, including a set of trocars and cannulas for sternal puncture, which I have used often.

7

WHAT OTHERS
THOUGHT OF HIM

I have collected the opinions of considerably more than 100 people who knew and worked with Bailey. They include his colleagues, assistants, anaesthetists, registrars, house surgeons, students, nurses, librarians, photographers, publishers, patients, and, most important of all, his widow.

It would be difficult to find any one about whom opinions were so varied, and I could easily fill this book three times with stories which I have been told about his tremendous enthusiasm for surgery, teaching ability, industry, kindness, moodiness, and intolerance of bores and incompetents.

I should hate anybody to say that I have 'whitewashed' Bailey, for many great men and women of the past are being debunked by the clever writers of today. I shall therefore start with the opinions expressed by one of his house surgeons who did not find him easy to work with:

'I was house surgeon at the Royal Northern Hospital to Sir Lancelot Barrington Ward, and for three months (I think August to October 1940) I was asked to fill in for his then house surgeon who had left through illness.

'I was very pleased to get the chance of working with such a man whose fame was then world-wide, and it was with mixed feelings that I first encountered him. I am 6 ft 4 in (the same height as Bailey) but I felt dwarfed and overpowered by what seemed to me a large gorilla.

'I had a very bad speech defect which has largely left me now, thank goodness, but he had no patience with it. It seemed impossible to carry on any conversation at ordinary levels. His mind moved so fast that I was left floundering. But one was borne along by his tremendous enthusiasm and the continuous excitement of his presence. I found myself neglecting Sir Lancelot and my other boss, Kenneth Walker, both quite patient and level-tempered.

'Ham seemed to live in a perpetual aura of crisis. We also had to contend with nightly air raids at that time, but this did not deter him. He did all his usual practice, which included a run down to Chatham Municipal Hospital on Saturdays, where he did a list of 13 or 14 cases straight off.

'You will probably know something of his operating methods, very speedy, frequent accidents. On the whole he might have been better sticking to writing his books, which were excellent in every way. But we in the house felt that in a serious case Ham might well get away with success. He was often very fast. I remember a simple mastectomy that I was rushing to towel up, and he rushed even faster and with two big knife strokes he had the breast off before I could even start putting towels on.

'We had several sharp disagreements. I fear I was not a very good house surgeon: frequent failures and omissions. I remember one such case when I was trying to say sorry and it would not come. We were on the stairs, and he kept climbing up to the top and climbing down again in a rage while I stood paralysed and speechless.

'Also, his dictaphone at home was disconcerting. He left a message via his secretary one evening with our night sister that he was not satisfied with my conduct of a certain case. I immediately rang the secretary who was a nice young lady.

'She said Mr Bailey was not in but would I like to say my piece into the dictaphone. So I did, and knowing he was not there I spoke perfectly and poured out a long list of complaints, ending up with, "It is also not usual to send serious complaints about one's house surgeon via the secretary". His only comment next day was, "You spoke well last night".

'It was a relief when his new house surgeon came into the house, an ex-boxer who could much better cope with him. I was left, perhaps not with love for his memory, but with great admiration for his drive, single-mindedness, and refusal to be deviated from the path that he had chosen. After his death I certainly rated him as the most memorable character with whom I was associated, ever.'

Nurses don't miss much. They notice all one's faults and remember them afterwards. I met many of Bailey's nurses. Though they remembered his faults, most of them seemed to like him and forgave him for them.

'Bailey was a remarkable man,' writes Sister M. L. who was with him at St Vincent's Clinic, 'with an infinite capacity for work. As the work increased he selected, when possible, colleagues imbued with the same ideals as himself. He instituted a follow-up clinic, making it available for the poor; indeed he spent a great deal of time looking for opportunities to render special help to such cases.

'A clear case of lack of means was to him like a clarion call to perform some extraordinary act of charity, and to such a call he would never turn a deaf ear. Quite often he gave to the Sister in Charge of the theatre money received for operations performed there to help buy necessary equipment. He had a strong weakness for helping those not blessed by a liberal share of worldly goods.'

Nurse C. of Potters Bar Hospital says, 'He was a very hardworking, genuine man, who lived for his work alone. He worked 18 hours out of 24 a day, but he was the most unpopular surgeon we ever had. He was not popular with the nurses or the doctors because he was a genius himself and had no time for anyone who was slow. When he came to see a patient he would expect you to have the whole story.

'He operated in the mornings on Thursdays and Saturdays. The patient had to be on the table at 8 a.m. Dr Elam, his anaesthetist, got on well with him. They could give one another cheek back. He always had a nurse to mop his head. She had to do it the proper way holding the towel in both hands. Just one swipe, no dabbing.

'If we wanted to know anything about a patient of Mr Bailey's we rang up Mrs Bailey and she would tell us. She was a charming person and always nice on the phone. Mr Bailey was always short. He was never nice. He didn't have time to be nice.'

A G.P. at Potters Bar said, 'He was a brilliant man but not the genial type that I like. He was like a calculating bit of machinery. You couldn't crack jokes with Hamilton Bailey. He lacked humanity; no joviality.'

At the Royal Northern I heard quite a different story from Sister W: 'I worked with him in the outpatients, operating theatre and wards. I loved him. He was grand to work with. We got on so well together, he and I. I was very fond of Hamilton. I helped him in his clinic in the out-patients from 1938 until he fell ill in 1948. He was efficient; he couldn't stand idiots; he liked everything to go with a swing. He was very kind to his patients and they liked him. They knew where they stood with him. Even now people still talk about him.

'He had quite a sense of humour. The first time I did his clinic I was not in tune with him. The next week he was not quite happy because he had lost his staff nurse. I told him, "The last staff nurse was with you for two years. I've been with you for two weeks." From that day we got on well. We worked very hard you know. Even during the war when the doodlebugs were dropping we went on just the same. He was kind to the nursing staff.'

Sister W. told me the story of how he had to have his head mopped when he was sweating. I have heard about his head-mopping from at least a dozen different sources. 'When he had the devil in him, if he turned to have his head mopped and you were not ready for him, he would turn back and say, "Too late".

'Some of the doctors were jealous. It was because of his efficiency. He used to dictate letters in his car when he left the hospital to the doctors who had sent in cases.'

Veta told me that Bailey had a great affection for Sister W. and thought she was an outstanding sister. She constantly demanded that she should go on working for Bailey although his out-patient sessions were probably much the busiest and hardest work. They made a good team.

Mr H. J. W., a member of the Friends' Ambulance Unit, a pacifist body formed to render medical service at home and abroad during the war, was based at one of the hospitals visited by Bailey at Chatham. 'The highlight of this work', he writes, 'was the visit each Monday by Mr Bailey, whom we knew as "Ham".

'I fancy his character had an element of the mischievous. One nurse, when asked to bring a piece of rubber tubing, probably allowed her haste to over-rule her judgement, and she brought a piece that was much too large. He told her that she should transfer to the fire service as she would be more at home among fire hoses.

'To another, who was unfortunate enough to break the silence by dropping some bowls, he suggested that a shooting gallery would be a more suitable place of employment for her. To those of us of the "section" this provided welcome light relief, something to be laughed at over the lunch table. Perhaps, not unnaturally, the nurses did not always see it that way.'

A lady clerk at the Royal Northern told me: 'He was just a big man in the distance. I was a junior clerk. Coming down the corridor he inspired awe. If you saw anyone running it was from fire, flood or Hamilton Bailey.'

At All Saints Hospital, Chatham, I heard yet another version of him, rather a midway assessment between his comparative unpopularity at Potters Bar and his near hero-worship at the Royal Northern. 'All the staff had the greatest respect for Hammy,' said Sister S. 'Everybody feared him. We were so scared that we took jolly good care we would get things right. One nurse was in tears nearly every time he came to the theatre, but she was the kind that never improved. He was unpopular with some nurses, but if you did your job well he was all right.'

Bailey's anaesthetists were often called upon to give anaesthetics for almost hopeless cases, for, perhaps on account of his acknowledged speed in operating, he was sometimes requested by his colleagues to operate on those whom most other surgeons of the day would be unwilling to tackle.

A radiotherapist told me that if a patient had a very large tumour which he didn't want to irradiate he would 'send it to Ham.' He was once known to remark to a nervous anaesthetist when the patient was not completely anaesthetised: 'I don't mind if they move; I don't mind if they vomit; as long as they don't complain of the technique!'

Dr Donald Blatchley, who gave many anaesthetics for him at the Royal Northern, told me: 'Ham had a reputation for eccentric behaviour in the operating theatre, but when one examines the things he did it can be seen that they were really for the benefit of the patient. All his funny ways were planned. He belonged to the generation of surgeons one of whose chief aims was speed in operating time. Nowadays, with improvements in anaesthesia and general care of the patient, surgery proceeds at a more leisurely speed.

'So he would not waste time by asking for things but developed a series of signals. For instance, when doing delicate plastic work on a kidney, at one stage in the procedure he would want to sit down. He would not remove his concentration from the operation to ask for a stool, but would do a little "knees bend" up and down until someone noticed. In those days we had solid square-topped stools, and he would continue his little jig until the stool was correctly placed so that he could feel the sides with his thighs, then he would sit down.

'He had a sure way of dealing with bureaucratic inefficiency. In the old days before autoclaves and pre-packed sterile instrument trays, at the Royal Northern the instruments were steam sterilised on the theatre premises. One day when I already had a patient – a simple mastectomy case, anaesthetised and on the table, Sister announced delay as there was no steam. "Send for the clerk of works", said Ham.

'This lone official had to deal with all the duties now divided and sub-divided among a host of civil servants. When he arrived, Ham took him by the shoulder to the theatre door, pointed to the patient and said, "See that poor woman being unnecessarily anaesthetised because your steam has failed? If anything happens I will go into the witness box and put the blame squarely on your shoulders." In no time we had a full head of steam.'

Dr John Elam, who anaesthetised for him at Potters Bar during the war and occasionally at the Royal Northern, writes: 'I did not like him at all at first but soon found that he had a heart of gold and did not know the meaning of the word jealousy. He did upset the nurses until they got to know him. He never minded what you said to him, and when the nurses got flustered I could always say, "Shut up, Ham" and he was all smiles.

'He liked to start his lists punctually at 8 a.m. so I had to get there at 7.30. This was before the relaxants came in, and he invariably wanted endotracheal ether (or chloroform when he was using diathermy). His great delight was the parotid tumour. He seemed to have one of these every week. He liked to do them on Saturday mornings as special cases.

'He would never despair of a patient and would tackle cases no one else would touch. I remember a man with a large abdominal mass which turned out to be a cancer invading coils of intestine: one would have thought a hopeless case. He removed it with sections of intestine, and was left with the task of restoring the continuity of the bowel by joining up the remaining portions in five places! The patient recovered and was going about Potters Bar ten years later.'

Dr J. L. B. writes, 'I knew Hamilton Bailey for many years during and after the second world war. I worked with him at St Vincent's Clinic and the Royal Northern, both as an anaesthetist and as his surgical assistant. He had an enormous capacity for work and it was not unusual for us to do up to 13 major operations a day, starting at 8 a.m. and carrying on until late evening.

'We never went out for meals and had sandwiches and tea sent up to the theatre. In addition, at the end of a long day's work he would record material for text books and articles. His style was so gripping that I labelled him the "Edgar Wallace of Surgery"! He had a most pleasing and affectionate personality, but his bedside manner was brusque, which did not always endear him to his patients, but he was a practical man and got on with the job. He never temporized. You either accepted his advice or went elsewhere.'

Dr R. C. writes, 'I knew Hamilton Bailey when I was a house

surgeon at the Royal Northern and he was at the peak of his powers. He was a very remarkable man with colossal energy and a wonderful teacher. I remember how on one occasion he came into the ward where one of my chief's patients was recovering from a complicated abdominal operation. He was being given a blood transfusion into one arm, having saline into the other arm, and receiving an intragastric milk drip. As he also had an infected bladder this was being irrigated with acriflavine, so that there were four bottles over the bed. This immediately caught Bailey's attention and he rushed out to his car and came back with a colour camera to record this unusual situation.'

Mr T. A. Nicholson, who worked for Bailey as a photographer for many years, told me how he started doing this work.

'I was with Topical Press Agency. I was specialising in railways, taking photographs of great locomotives and things. I didn't know anything about surgery. Then, one day, I got a note asking me to go out to the Consolation Hospital. It was there that I first met Hamilton Bailey. He was going to do a thyroidectomy, and he wanted me to take "stills" of various stages of the operation.

'He said, "Are you ready?" I had my camera arranged in the right place. Then he seemed to cut the man's head off. He made an incision right across the neck. It was a bit of a shock because I had never seen an operation before. He stopped the bleeding with forceps, then stood aside. "Photograph it," he said.

'When he'd finished the session of operations and I had taken several more photographs he said, "We're looking for a photographer. You're number six, the first that's walked out. The others had all apparently fainted and been carried out.

'So that was how he took me on. I got the contract for Topical Press at the Royal Northern Hospital. Bailey started the photographic department there.

'Any interesting case was photographed. In the out-patients department when Bailey wanted a patient photographed he would ask him to wait outside. I remember up to eight of them waiting to be photographed. I'd hear them saying to one another, "How much longer is he going to be?".

'Bailey always knew exactly what he wanted. All we had to do was to take the pictures. "How much film have you got?" he would ask when, for example, he was going to take a stone out of a kidney. "Go and sit there. Get your camera and lights fixed here, and be ready. Now this is what I'm going to do . . .

' "Are you ready? Now we are going to take 30 ft". He'd tell you what angle to set your camera. When he'd finished the operation, with no mistakes, and you'd used up exactly the amount of film needed, he came out of the theatre and gave *you* full credit for making the film. Then you'd send him a bill for taking it. When you mentioned this he said, "It's very valuable film. How else can I get it?".'

Mr Nicholson said, 'Sometimes he'd ring up asking for a photo. He'd say, "I want that one of the kidney stones with the ruler placed alongside (to show the reader of his books the size of the stones). Can you find it? All right, bring it along." Whatever time it was I'd have to go straight out to Totteridge with the films. He'd say "All right, I want that one. Have some slides ready in the morning." He would need slides when he gave lectures.

'Then Mrs Bailey would come in and ask if I had eaten any supper. I'd reply, "He hasn't given me a chance." So Mrs Bailey would get me something to eat. Bailey and his wife were a terrific team.

'In the theatre at Consolation, Bailey would stick out his hand for an instrument. If they gave him the wrong instrument he was annoyed. He seemed to think that the sister could thought-read what he wanted. Afterwards he would be sorry for his annoyance. The important thing for him was the patient. It wouldn't matter whether the patient could pay or not.

'One day, when he was annoyed with the sister handing him the instruments, another sister, a nun, touched his arm and said, "If you could operate as well as that sister can give you instruments the patient would have nothing to worry about." After that he never complained to the instrument sister.'

Mr L. T. Clifford, Bailey's other photographer who became Nicholson's partner, was concerned with the movie films. He told me how greatly impressed he was with Bailey's memory. 'While working on a film of the parotid gland we first sat down and projected the film in rough form. Mr Bailey made notes of what he wanted done, and he asked me to have the film ready in about six weeks.

'While I was preparing the film I scratched it a bit, but I thought I could get round this by cutting the film. It was a portion showing a section of the jaw. I reassembled it and had it ready on the appointed date.

'He saw the film through, then got up very quietly and sat beside me. He repeated his original instructions precisely from memory and let me know that he wasn't to be trifled with. I apologised and did the film the way he wanted it.

'During the months that we worked with him he wanted to know all about tape recorders, which were just coming in. They were big, clumsy things then and cost about £360. He visualised the possibility of sending the tapes to other countries.

'If he had been in any other sphere, with his drive he would have gone a long way. He had such a brilliant brain.'

One of his patients, Mrs R., writes, 'My doctor sent me to see Mr Hamilton Bailey in 1937 at the Royal Northern, Holloway. I was treated by him for a considerable time in the out-patients department, after which I went to him at intervals for examinations until around 1943. After this I went to St Vincent's Clinic where he continued to see me until he had to give up, and Mr Swain took over from him.

'I understand that I was in a very bad way when I first went to Mr Bailey. My own doctor told me that the treatment was equal to a major operation, so I have much to be thankful for. He was a very kindly man and I was deeply sorry to hear of his death.'

I met Mrs R. and also Mr Swain, from whom I discovered that Mrs R. was treated for tumours of the bladder by electrocoagulation of the tumours through a cystoscope. When I saw her in 1970 she was perfectly well.

Another of his patients did not seem so pleased with him. She was a private patient at St Vincent's Clinic on whom Bailey had

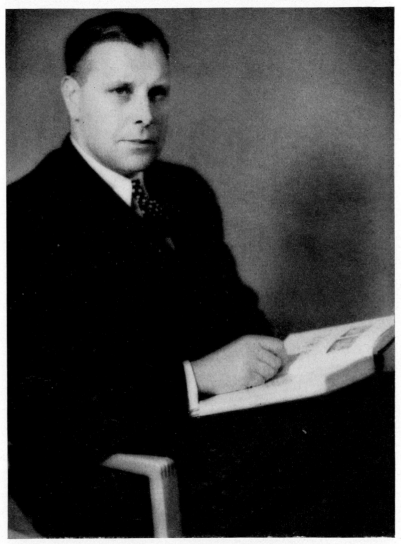

7. Hamilton Bailey, aged 33.

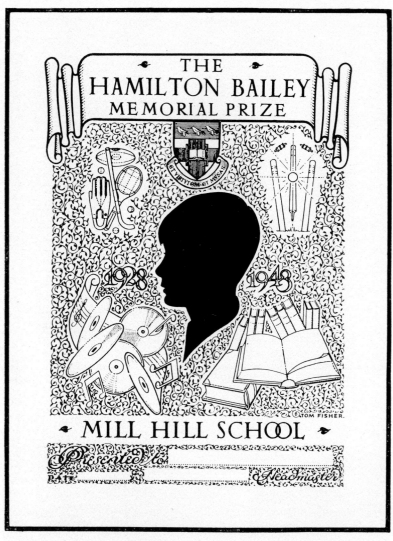

8. Book plate designed by Bailey in memory of his son who died in 1943, aged 15.

performed the operation of hysterectomy during the war. She complained that Bailey came to see her after the operation only once or twice, and that she was unwell for some time afterwards. This lady, on whom I called at her London flat in 1970, was not one of his poorer patients.

Dr K., whom I knew in 1933 while we were both assistant medical officers at Hope Hospital, Salford, told me how, while doing a locum in Birmingham, he developed a whitlow of his left hand. Having read *Physical Signs*, he decided to consult Bailey, who welcomed him at his home. Dr K. wrote in answer to my request in 1970 for the detailed story; 'He suggested that I foment the hand as it was not quite ready for incision. However, with a little persuasion he agreed to incise. He took me in his car to the hospital. He incised the indurated area: no pus. Saline soaks eased the discomfort.

'My impressions of Bailey: a pleasant and agreeable man, kindly and easy to talk to. He laughed readily. When I saw him he had been writing. During our conversation I happened to mention his book on physical signs. His face lit up; he laughed and was in great form.'

8

BAILEY'S OTHER BOOKS

In 1932, soon after Bailey's arrival at the Royal Northern Hospital, he and Love produced the first edition of their book, *Short Practice of Surgery*. Their collaboration was comparable with that of Gilbert and Sullivan. Though Bailey and Love worked at the same hospital they did not often meet, and much of their communication was done by post but, as with Gilbert and Sullivan, the result was successful and the book passed through its many editions and reprints with applause from the reviewers of most medical journals.

I could find only one journal which gave unfavourable criticism of one edition: the fourth. This was *Guy's Hospital Gazette*, which devoted 1,300 words to a wholesale condemnation of the book, except for the quality of the illustrations and the paper and binding of the publishers. It concluded the review with a warning to students to avoid the book:

'Like the devil incarnate, its outward appearance is good, but it must inevitably lead to disaster.'

Bailey thought that the reference to the devil incarnate would be good copy for advertising the book, and persuaded the publishers, who agreed with reluctance to insert whole page advertisements in the *British Medical Journal* and *Guy's Hospital Gazette* quoting the words of the review. After this it continued to sell better than ever.

Love was not Bailey's only collaborator with whom communications were conducted predominantly by post; there were many others. Indeed one of his most valued colleagues with whom he corresponded for 17 years, met him only once. This was Mr Francis Bauer of Liverpool. Their co-operation started at the end

37

of the war when, after reading *Physical Signs,* Mr Bauer sent Bailey some suggestions concerning differential diagnosis of various ear diseases.

Bailey's response was enthusiastic, and he asked Bauer to review some of his other books, supply clinical photographs, and eventually to contribute chapters on ear, nose and throat conditions for *Demonstrations of Operative Surgery* and *Emergency Surgery.* Over the years Bauer and Bailey exchanged scores of letters, but they met personally only once in 1948. Bauer was attending a lecture by an American ear specialist in London, and stayed overnight with Bailey.

Bailey wrote three books for nurses, for whom, despite his bullying tactics, he felt great affection and sympathy. The first was a joint work by Bailey and Love, entitled *Surgery for Nurses.* It was published in 1933, and went into nine editions, but when Bailey became ill in 1948 he was unable to continue revising it. The subsequent editions lacked his magical touch, and the last edition was in 1964.

His second book for nurses was *101 Clinical Demonstrations for Nurses,* of which there were only two editions, in 1944 and 1946. For some unfathomable reason it failed to sell as well as his other books. It was his last book for nurses, *Demonstrations of Operative Surgery,* intended to interest also general practitioners and students, which was in my opinion the best. This first appeared in 1945, and was edited by Bailey, who asked many leading authorities to contribute. The last edition was published in 1967, revised by Mr A. R. Isaac. Bailey also edited and contributed articles to *Nursing Illustrated,* born 1938 and incorporated in *Nursing Mirror* in 1941.

Two books by Bailey were published in 1936: *Diseases of the Testicle,* and, in collaboration with Norman Matheson, *Recent Advances in Genito-Urinary Surgery. Clinical Surgery for Dental Practitioners* appeared in 1937, and in 1938 he edited the 11th edition of *Pye's Surgical Handicraft,* first published in 1884 by Walter Pye. Only two editions had appeared in the previous 20 years before Bailey became editor but now new editions appeared, eight in 15 years, each better and more profusely illustrated than the last, and circulation rapidly increased.

When the war came, an authoritative work on war surgery was urgently needed for, apart from several excellent books on fractures, there was no book to serve the needs of surgeons coping with battle casualties. The publishers, E. & S. Livingstone of Edinburgh, Scotland, were the first to realise the growing demand for such a book. Mr Charles Macmillan of Livingstone's thought that there was only one man in the country who could undertake this colossal task and do it expeditiously.

Mr Macmillan has told me that he was always attracted to Bailey as an outstanding medical author. He was impressed by the sensation caused by John Wright & Sons when they published *Demonstrations of Physical Signs in Clinical Surgery*, for the author was then unknown.

Mr Macmillan writes, 'But his superb illustrations at once stamped this book as a "classic". Later on, the same firm published *Emergency Surgery*. This authoritative work which met a great need was also an outstanding success. Two books published by H. K. Lewis I envied: *Short Practice of Surgery* and *Surgery for Nurses*.

'I simply longed to meet and get to know this amazing medical author. I used to watch him when his car was held up in London's busy traffic. He worked hard between appointments, either private or at various hospitals so widely scattered where he was on the staff.

'Oblivious to what was happening in the busy streets or in the country lanes he could be seen working on his dictaphone which was suitably installed in his spacious Rolls-Royce. Every day he must write something. He always set himself a target which he usually attained by sheer determined discipline.

'Both Mr Hamilton Bailey and his wife were enthusiastic about our proposition. Within a few months a team of contributors was arranged, and the first part of about 128 pages was on sale. Hard work was involved, but it was a magnificent publishing achievement.

'During the war years on many occasions while the city was frequently bombed I stayed at his lovely home in Totteridge. In our discussions I learned the secret of his success as a medical author. The presentation must be perfect and lavishly illustrated.

'After the typists' work from the dictaphone reels was completed, and perhaps retyped many times, next day's task would be carefully considered and arranged in advance. The important feature in all the books was the illustrations. No expense was spared: only the best was good enough for Bailey. The line drawings must be perfect in every detail. The lettering on the drawing was planned so that no essential detail was hidden from view.'

Surgery of Modern Warfare was certainly edited under the right conditions, because most of it was done during the active bombing of London. Bailey and Veta sat in their raid shelter at Denham, their first house at Totteridge, with the aircraft guns booming and the bombs falling.

There were 65 contributors in the first edition which came out in 1941, 72 in the second, and 77 in the third. An examination of the manuscripts has shown me how much Bailey did to clarify and re-arrange the material of some of the contents in his performance of the colossal task.

I have mentioned all but one of Bailey's books; this was *Notable Names in Medicine and Surgery*, which he wrote in collaboration with Mr W. J. Bishop, the librarian of the Royal Society of Medicine. It was the only one of his books which was not of practical use to surgeons or nurses, but despite this limitation it went into three editions and has just been revised. He also contributed to *The Royal Northern Operative Surgery*, second edition, in 1951, and edited the Genito-Urinary Section of the *Medical Annual* from 1933 to 1948, the last contribution being completed by Mr Norman Matheson while Bailey was ill.

9

LONDON AND OVERWORK

In January 1931 Bailey went to London where he joined the staff of the Royal Northern Hospital. Mr Love was elected at the same time. Six years after they were rejected by the London Hospital, the Royal Northern had now appointed two of the most prominent surgeons of the century.

Bailey hoped for an appointment on the staff of a London undergraduate teaching hospital. He applied to some of them without success, and quite late in his career (in 1946) he was apparently still hankering after a teaching hospital, for at the comparatively advanced age of 51 he applied for the Chair of Surgery in Cape Town. Dr Cole Rous was the successful applicant.

Bailey however was accepted by numerous other hospitals. At various times between 1931 and 1948 he worked at a dozen or more. One of these was the Italian Hospital, a Roman Catholic institution, which was closed down in 1941. The Sisters of Charity of St Vincent de Paul who staffed it decided to replace it by the St Vincent's Clinic in Ladbroke Grove, Notting Hill, and asked Bailey to help them. Bailey, an atheist, was highly regarded by the nuns at St Vincent's and for a long time was the only surgeon there. He often operated for nothing and paid the fees for the bed and the anaesthetists of patients who could not afford them. Before the inauguration of the National Health Service there were many patients who needed such help, e.g. elderly spinsters with Graves's disease. I have listened to glowing accounts of Bailey's help to patients treated at this clinic, which was spoken of by many as the 'Hamilton Bailey Clinic'.

Bailey started his duties at the Royal Northern while still working in Bristol. From his operation books I found that he was still operating at the Homeopathic Hospital in Bristol right up to 19

February 1931 though he started at the Royal Northern on 9 January when he performed an excision of the ear for cancer on a woman aged 81 and four other operations. He must have made several journeys between the two cities from 3 January to 20 February, for between these dates he completed seven sessions in the operating theatre at Bristol as well as seven in London.

During his first year at the Royal Northern, his income from private practice was a bare £300. In 'Black November' of 1931 he came home at the end of the month depressed after a day of interviewing lay committees in search of another hospital appointment. His total earnings for November were nil, there was not one 3-guinea consultation, but it was the sense of failure rather than the lack of money which upset him.

During his second year at the Royal Northern his income reached £1,800. He never charged astronomical fees. Veta cannot remember him receiving as much as 100 guineas from more than five patients for any operation. His usual fee for appendicectomy was 25 guineas. Now the operation costs between £50 and £70.

Veta used to ring up the doctor who sent the patient to ask what fee he or she considered that the patient could pay. If the patient could not afford to pay a moderately reduced fee he often charged practically nothing. He was interested only in doing the work.

It will be wondered how it was that Bailey, who was so generous to vast numbers of patients, casual about obtaining fees, and treated most of his patients at the hospital for nothing, ever made his practice pay. The explanation was that he was extremely good at his work and took a great deal of trouble to give his patients the best he could. He had the biggest operating lists and the largest number of out-patients at the Royal Northern and at most of the other hospitals he attended.

The patients came to him because they thought he was a good surgeon; certainly not for his bedside manner, which was non-existent. The doctors sent him patients because he was efficient in dealing with them and sent them reports. In other words, Bailey was successful because of his skill and industry.

Bailey and Veta first went to live at Hendon in a three-bed-roomed semi-detached house given to Veta by Bailey's father. They sold it after 18 months and bought a larger detached house at Mill Hill where they remained for four years. Bailey took consulting rooms at 35 Harley Street.

From Mill Hill they moved to Denham in Totteridge, where they remained for many years. It was here that Bailey installed a swimming pool, a converted tuberculosis hut, dictaphones, telephone recorder, and other gadgets.

The tremendous array of paraphernalia which he built up over the years was designed to enable him to do the maximum possible amount of work, to occupy every moment of the day usefully, and to waste no time. His eagerness to achieve his object caused him to overlook one thing: the limit to which the human frame can be subjected. He always overworked. When Bailey and Veta went for a holiday it was not a holiday; they went loaded up with trunks of manuscripts, photographs, x-rays, and other equipment. Bailey did not know how to relax.

His hobbies, if such they could be called, were all designed to keep him fit rather than to provide rest. He played quite good golf (handicap 11), most often with Veta (handicap 9), but there was always someone at the club-house to wave a white towel telling him to come back if he was wanted on the telephone.

He used to play golf with Dr George A. Shepherd, a general practitioner with whom he was friendly, at Hadley Wood, where Bailey was a member. He never used a wooden club; he was not steady with it, and he told Dr Shepherd, 'I hate to do anything that I don't do well.' He used a number one iron from the tees.

After the game they would go and have one drink and a little chat at the club-house, but Bailey never talked much, and then only about his work and his books. He talked little about himself. He practised his golf on his small six-hole golf course at home. He also did a little trout and salmon fishing. His favourite exercise was swimming.

For obtaining the maximum efficiency he gradually developed

his massive organisation with three resident secretaries. This took several years. He slept in a converted tuberculosis hut in the garden, one side of which was completely open to provide plenty of fresh air. It could be rotated to ensure protection at all times from the prevailing wind. He started work at 5 a.m. While lying in bed for a bit he would work with his dictaphone, then get up and make a pot of tea. Then he would have a swim. The gardener would come and help him to break the ice sometimes in the winter, for it could be cold at Totteridge.

Mr Macmillan said while staying with Bailey he felt compelled to get up and join him in the pool, for Bailey laid out a pair of swimming trunks and a towel for him when he heard his friend liked a morning swim. Afterwards Bailey produced a large, heavy medicine ball. 'You had to be fit,' said Mr Macmillan, 'to withstand his vigorous onslaught.

'On such an occasion his young son, Hamilton, joined us. For some time he stood there shivering at the water's edge. It seemed to take a lot of courage on his part to take the plunge. I asked him if he liked it. He answered emphatically, "No, I hate it". I asked him why he did it. He replied, "Got to. If you really knew the Guv'nor you'd understand." He gave me such a sly look as much as to say, "You are only a guest and see what you *have* to see".'

After the swim Bailey went to his bathroom, converted from part of the stables. There he might have a Turkish bath but often he did not allow himself time, for one of his anaesthetists told me that Bailey would arrive in the winter mornings blue from the swimming pool. The bath was followed by an alcohol rub-down and a shave.

At 7.45 he came into the house for breakfast, and then off to work before 8 a.m. During that last few minutes three items – a gold cigarette case, lighter, and a pencil on a chain – were occasionally mislaid, although he was habitually tidy.

'And what a hunt it was,' Veta told me, 'three secretaries, the cook, the housemaid and I, all looking. I well remember the sigh of relief when the car actually moved off on these occasions. While he was eating his breakfast I was taking down instructions for the work of the day for the secretaries. He always dealt with them through me.'

When Bailey first started to use mechanical means of dictating he used dictaphones; the recording was done on wax cylinders. He had one in his garden hut, one in his car, one in his study, and one attached to his telephone at Totteridge with which a record could automatically be kept of conversations about his patients and of information useful for compiling his books.

This device was installed before the war, and I believe that there were only two similar gadgets in London at this time (one being at the Soviet Embassy). The words spoken were recorded on a revolving drum, and the instrument could be switched on and off as desired by a lever next to the phone. The machine was large, requiring a table to itself.

He used the dictaphone in his Rolls-Royce for recording material for books or notes on patients. After his morning session at the first hospital out-patient department, he would dictate letters to doctors who had sent him patients giving results of his clinical findings. Later he would dictate letters to the same doctors telling them the results of any x-rays or other investigations. After driving him to the next hospital, his chauffeur would take the dictaphone records back to Totteridge, where his secretaries typed the letters, which Bailey would check and sign that night.

By the time he had finished his work at the second hospital, the chauffeur would be back to drive him to Harley Street. Then the Rolls would return to Totteridge with the drum containing the second set of reports on patients.

A general practitioner who referred patients to Bailey told me, 'I'd send a patient to his out-patient department. The very next day I'd receive a letter from him saying, "Thank you for the notes on Mrs so-and-so. Such-and-such investigations are being done." Later on he'd send me the results of the investigations. By doing this he built up a tremendous consulting practice. He was very popular with his patients and very kind to them indeed.

'He often came on domiciliary visits. He was excellent at that. I never saw him lose his temper. He was irritable at times in the theatre if the nurses didn't work well. He had an impulsive nature, but more so in the theatre – never in making a diagnosis. He was an excellent operator: quick, but gentle with the abdominal organs.'

I suggested that there was some disagreement about his operative skill, to which the G.P. replied, 'I assisted him with many operations, and he was absolutely first class.'

On reaching home in the evening he would resume work on his books and articles. He was often called at night for emergencies, and would think nothing of travelling 60 miles or so to operate at some country hospital.

During the war, Bailey rang up the petroleum officer to ask for extra coupons. Living at Totteridge, which is some distance away from London but well situated for visiting the country hospitals to which his patients were admitted, his cars consumed a good deal of petrol, especially when he was particularly busy.

The petroleum officer was not impressed with Bailey's reason for his need for additional coupons, and asked why he could not call a taxi. Bailey explained that the nearest taxi rank was at Golders Green about five miles away, and it was difficult to get a taxi in the middle of the night, but the official refused the coupons. A record of this conversation was taken on the dictaphone.

Bailey wrote a letter to a medical journal complaining he would be considerably delayed in reaching an emergency case in the middle of the night because his coupons would be exhausted before the end of the month. His letter was quoted in the lay press.

Soon afterwards, Bailey received a telephone call from the Minister responsible for rationing petrol. This conversation was similarly recorded on the dictaphone. The Minister complained that Bailey was libelling his department. He was quite certain, he remarked, that the petroleum officer would not refuse coupons to a doctor needing them. Bailey then invited him to listen to the record which he had of his conversation with the petroleum officer. On receiving this unexpected invitation, the Minister apologised, and after that there was no more trouble about petrol.

Later, when tape recorders came in, Bailey switched to those.

He had two large machines and one of pocket size. This last he used to take with him to the British Medical Association Library where Mr T. John Shields, the librarian, would have prepared the piles of journals which he needed in a private room. Then, instead of making notes, Bailey dictated all references and articles into the tape recorder, which Veta transcribed next day.

The tape recorder was a great time-saver but it could not have been used without the co-operation of Mr Shields, who provided a private room, for Bailey would not have been able to talk into a machine in one of the library's public rooms.

When Bailey and Veta went on a trip to Europe he left his telephone number with his secretaries so that he could be called back if any of his patients required attention. He once performed a prostatectomy on the morning of the day on which he and Veta flew to Switzerland. This was perhaps unwise, for of all the operations done in surgery, removal of the prostate gland is one of those most likely to give trouble during the post-operative period. The prostatic bed may bleed; the catheter may get blocked with blood clot; infection may supervene; or the patient may suffer from post-operative shock. Many surgeons do not like to leave the after-care to a colleague.

When they arrived in Berne he received a telephone call telling him that the patient was not doing well, and he and Veta flew home immediately. The holiday was abandoned, but not in vain, for the patient recovered.

Just after the last war, Bailey visited the U.S.A. on a lecture tour. He was invited to come for a restful week-end at a log cabin in Canada. On the way to the cabin, a luxurious building where there was little of the quiet fishing for which it was allegedly used, his host remarked casually that he had promised to take Bailey to give a lecture to some post-graduates in London, Ontario.

During the journey, a surgeon sitting next to Bailey at the back of the car remarked that nursing in the United States was on the downgrade, and he asked Bailey what the nursing was like in England. Bailey made some non-committal reply to the effect that, considering that the war was only just over, and the demand for nurses in the fighting forces considerable, they got on very well. In truth, Bailey had the highest opinion of British nurses, though he was certainly inclined to bully them when they were inefficient at some of the hospitals.

At the post-graduate meeting, the surgeon who had been travelling with Bailey spoke to a woman reporter sitting next to him about the way nursing in the United States was deteriorating. He implied that his friend, Hamilton Bailey, who was lecturing, had mentioned that the same thing was happening in England. The reporter wrote an article for her newspaper saying Bailey had remarked on the inferior quality of nursing in England. Bailey knew nothing about this, but the item was quoted widely in the British press, implying that Bailey had made a speech in Ontario decrying British nurses.

Reporters rang up Veta in England, asking what she knew about it. Disturbed, she sent a cable to Bailey with the words, 'Make no more reference to nurses.' Bailey was naturally perplexed when he received the cable in Chicago, for he could not remember having referred to nurses at all. He was so worried about it that he sat through a performance of 'Oklahoma', to which he had been taken by Max Thorek, and could remember nothing of it afterwards.

Dr Thorek was the founder of the International College of Surgeons, with its headquarters in Chicago. It was I think the only surgical institution dear to Bailey's heart. He contributed as much as, if not more than, any other British surgeon to the International College, of which he became an honorary Fellow and Vice President in 1947.

During his career as a surgeon Bailey became a member of numerous societies, colleges and associations, but he seldom attended their meetings. He took particular interest only in the International College. This interest probably started in October 1938, when he wrote an article in the first volume of the Transactions of the International College of Surgeons on the transverse upper abdominal incision. After that he contributed 19 more articles to the journal.

Why he became so attached to this College I cannot say for sure, but I think it was because Bailey was more greatly appreciated abroad (through his writings) than in Britain. This bears out Christ's words quoted in St Mark, ch.6, v.4, that 'a prophet is not without honour, save in his own country, and among his own kin, and in his own house.'

In Britain he made many enemies. He held strong views which, because they did not always agree with those of his contemporaries, aroused enmity. He was supremely successful at his medical writing from a comparatively early age, which brought him many admirers, and he soon became an authority on the art of diagnosis.

Most of his students greatly admired him and he was adored by many young surgeons working under him, but some of his chiefs and contemporaries became his jealous opponents. He apparently cared little about what anybody thought of him. Though a victim of jealousy, he was never jealous himself; indeed he was tolerant of his enemies.

It would be impossible to become a successful surgeon without arousing admiration among those who benefit from one's skill and industry. Similarly, the writer of surgical text books who imparts his knowledge as accurately, clearly and impressively, as Bailey did, could not fail to become well known. Only those in competition with him or who disliked him would refuse recognition.

Surgery and surgical writing cannot be carried out anonymously. Success in both these arts usually involves benefit to the human race, which may be one of the reasons why surgery is so popular a profession.

Bailey became famous, and through his writings will become more so, but with some of those who counted he was never recognised. There is no painted portrait of Bailey in any of the Royal Colleges or in any Royal Society. He was never admitted to the staff of any undergraduate teaching hospital except one at Liverpool where he was so thwarted by his opponents that he soon shook the dust of it off his feet.

In the British Commonwealth outside Britain and in foreign countries Bailey was appreciated, because his books were so useful:

in Britain he was regarded by his seniors as a competitor. But at the Royal Northern, where they knew him best, his work was recognised, as evidenced by the establishment of a little museum in his memory and by the recent opening of a new operating theatre in St David's Wing dedicated as a tribute to him.

Bailey had a rooted objection to doing anything which he regarded as a waste of time. He seldom went to theatres, dances, or formal dinners. He had no love for music, but he liked pictures and poetry. He seldom read a book outside of surgery, medicine and related subjects, and could discuss few subjects other than these. But he could quote extensively from the Bible, though he did not believe in any god.

Yet some people who were his direct antithesis got on well with him. Dr J. L. Hopkins, who gave anaesthetics for him, was a Welshman whose great interest was race horses. He was a fanatical punter. He even got the nuns at St Vincent's Clinic and the Consolation Hospital betting on horses, a complete contrast to Bailey.

Bailey did not like driving; hence his chauffeur. Veta maintains that he was quite a good driver, but apt to wait for the green to turn red before driving on at intersections! A less biased observer, a porter at the Royal Northern, has told me that Bailey was a 'terrible driver.'

Bailey enjoyed his food. He had a special fancy for seagull's eggs. A mystical belief has somehow circulated among readers of books that when an author has a book published the publisher takes the author out to lunch; an attractive but erroneous belief. Even Bailey, who got on well with his publishers, was never wined, dined, or even lunched by any of them.

He liked a whisky and soda at night, but never drank to excess. He smoked about 20 cigarettes a day. He could not get on with a pipe, for he bit through the stem, and did not care for cigars.

Bailey dressed well; almost all his clothes were specially made for him. His size 8 gloves had to be made for him because of the missing finger, and also his size 12 shoes because he suffered from deformities of his feet accentuated by his badly-fitting boots at school. He wore a jewelled gold tie pin which ruined his shirts and

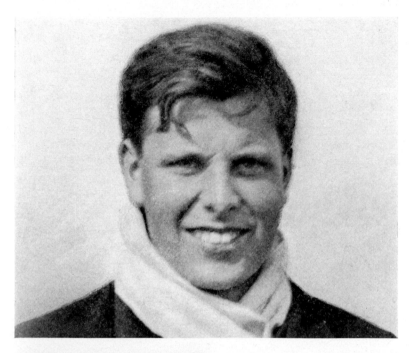

9. Young Bailey, serving in the Navy.

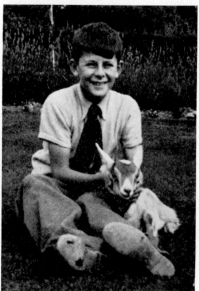

10. His son Hamilton with the pet kid which he delivered from its mother.

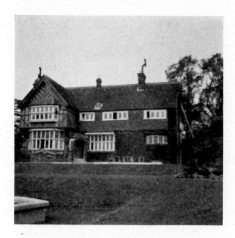

11. Bailey's first house at Totteridge common. It was in one of the cottages adjoining that the editorial offices of *Nursing Illustrated* were sited.

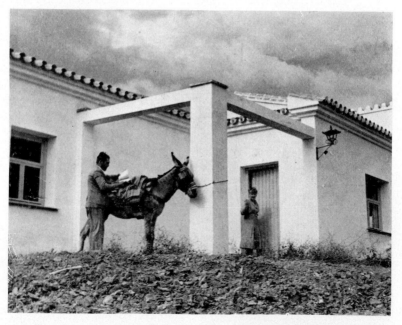

12. The post arrives at Bailey's last home in Fuengirola, Spain, in 1960.

ties. His Savile Row outfit was I think an unconscious rebellion against his parents who had grossly neglected his dress in childhood.

He liked a close shave and was meticulous about cleanliness. Apart from his morning bath he took a Turkish bath every Friday while working in London when he could fit it in between his operating sessions. As he got older and took less exercise his weight rose from 14½ stone to about 17 stone, but he was never a fat man, as he was so tall.

So intense was Bailey's dislike of formality that he never once attended a ceremonial dinner at the Royal College of Surgeons. The number of occasions during his married life on which he donned evening dress probably did not go into double figures. The only kind of evening entertainment which he enjoyed outside his own home was going out to dinner at least once a week with Veta.

He was a very shy man, who did not like publicity. Sometimes he held parties at his house which were attended by doctors from all over the world. He liked doing this, but found them an ordeal.

His favourite pets were the tropical fish in electrically-heated tanks in his study at home and in his consulting rooms. He said he liked them because they were colourful and did not make a noise. Yet at Totteridge, with his contradictory nature, he had a pet dog of which he was fond, which must have been noisy unless it was exceptional. It was sold to him as a smooth-haired Shetland sheep dog but its parentage was doubtful. He also liked Siamese cats: the noisiest of the feline family.

During the war they had four lambs, one of which Veta sent to the slaughter-house because they were short of meat while their son, Hamilton, was at home for the school holidays. After they had all enjoyed a lavish supply of meat for six days, both Bailey and his son became uneasy. 'This isn't ours, is it?' one of them asked. When Veta admitted that it was their own lamb neither of them would eat another bite.

10

'HAM' REACHES
BREAKING POINT

Young Hamilton, their only child, was born in Birmingham on 16 April 1928. From the time of his birth he was an extremely well-behaved child. Veta remembers having to get up to attend to him at night only once since he was born.

As they moved afterwards from place to place, he grew up as a normal and intelligent child. Most of Veta's time was occupied in helping Bailey with the preparation of his first book, and it seems today surprising that out of Bailey's meagre salary they succeeded in employing a maid and a nanny to help look after the baby.

When he started going to school he was an outstanding pupil and a keen sportsman. He excelled at cricket. He was moreover a remarkably happy boy who seemed to inherit from his father a complete disregard for money. If his mother forgot to give him his pocket money he would forget to ask for it.

He was educated at a preparatory school in Kent, then at Mill Hill School, a few miles from his home in Totteridge. He was quiet, thoughtful and well-mannered, with a keen sense of fun, a gay and happy temperament, full of zest and enthusiasm for everything he undertook, and utterly devoted to his mother, whom he closely resembled both in appearance and character. On one occasion, while his parents were away from home, he received news that he had received eight credits in an examination, and his one thought was to tell his mother the good news. Bailey took little interest in his son or in his progress at school.

Young Hamilton was a good swimmer, and a daily dip in the swimming pool was a regular routine when he was at home for the holidays. Even when the ice had to be removed from the top of the pool he would faithfully follow his father in, albeit reluctantly on the coldest days.

When the flying bombs started to fall in London, young Hamilton's school was moved to St Bees in Cumberland. It was while the boy was coming home from school on 29 July 1943 that death struck suddenly and unexpectedly. At Preston, while the train was stationary he leant out of the window of the railway carriage. As a train went past a door swung open; it hit him on the head, instantly killing him.

Veta, on hearing the shocking news, rang up Potters Bar Hospital, where Bailey was operating, and asked a senior member of the staff to inform him as soon as he had finished the operation which he was doing. Instead, the person to whom Veta spoke went straight to the theatre and blurted out the news in the middle of an operation for removal of the gall bladder. He had to finish as there was not even a house surgeon there.

As he said to Veta afterwards, 'My mind went completely numb. I told myself that I must be extra careful.' When he had finished the operation successfully, he wrote the patient up for half a pint of blood. Though the donor's and recipient's bloods were correctly grouped and cross-matched, a severe reaction followed, and the patient died.

Bailey blamed himself bitterly for the transfusion reaction. To the distress resulting from his son's death was added the self-recrimination for a transfusion reaction resulting from the administration of blood which he had ordered, 'to be extra careful'.

Bailey, who no doubt reproached himself for neglecting the boy, was never the same after this dual disaster. While most men would have been able to resort to outside interests to take their minds off their grief, Bailey had none. He could not divert his mind with a detective story, a visit to the theatre, an exciting game of chance or a relaxing holiday. Golf would be of little use to one seeking relief from despondency. His only interest was his work, at which he drove himself harder than ever.

A G. P., who knew Bailey well at the Royal Northern, recalled to me, 'When I went to hospital the following morning, Sister McClusky was on duty. I was shocked when she told me about Bailey's son. While I was talking to her Bailey arrived in the ward. When I told him how sorry I was, he couldn't speak. He put his hands over his eyes.

'That night I went to see them at their house in Totteridge. I told the maid who I was and asked her to tell them that I had called but that I wouldn't come up unless they wanted to see me. She came back and told me that they did, so I went up and sat with them for the best part of a couple of hours. I felt my visit had done them some good, persuading him that he still had something to live for.'

Veta told me years afterwards how glad they were to see this man who tried to comfort them. He struck me as the kind of man whose sympathy and understanding would help anyone similarly placed. But Bailey had few other friends to comfort him. He was indeed a lone wolf, liked and admired by many but with only his wife close enough to him to understand him; and Veta too was stricken with grief.

After his son's death Bailey insisted that all traces of him should be obliterated from their house, presumably so that he would not be constantly reminded of the boy which would activate his guilt complex. Each year, as the anniversary of little Hamilton's death approached he became more irritable and restless, and hardly slept at all. The ordeal through which Veta passed during this period can hardly be imagined until, in 1948, Bailey suffered a mental breakdown.

Considering the family history of mental instability which affected both his mother and his sister, it is not surprising that Bailey himself became affected. It is possible that his insanity was inevitable but its onset was undoubtedly precipitated by his son's death, and perhaps more so by his reaction to it. It took the form of a manic-depressive psychosis.

During the summer of 1948 he became irritable and excited, with delusions, for which he was confined to a mental institution.

He partially recovered during 1949–51 after 22 electroconvulsant treatments. While living at home he remained constantly depressed, frightened, and unable to sleep, but sufficiently improved to revise *Short Practice of Surgery*.

In 1951, when he relapsed, he was again admitted to a mental hospital – this time at Graylingwell, Chichester, on an Urgency Order, suffering from mania. There was no specific treatment for mania in those days; he was treated with sedatives and electroconvulsive therapy, but without effect. During 1952 there was no improvement – if anything he was worse, and leucotomy, the last resort for treating uncontrollable patients, was considered. His wife and friends began to fear that he would never improve.

In 1953, an Australian psychiatrist, David Moore, advised the use of lithium carbonate, with which treatment was started on 7 October 1953. There was an immediate improvement, but he relapsed again in November.

Mr Bauer, valued contributor to some of his books, was one of the few who remained confident that Bailey would recover. When Bailey was better he wrote to Bauer: 'Please remember I am very grateful to you, perhaps more than to any other, for the enormous assistance you have given me in stimulus and knowledge far beyond the scope of your special subject.'

Veta went to the north of England for Christmas 1953, where she endured the festival under depressing circumstances with her aged and sick parents, both discussing their real and imaginary ailments, and with the news of her husband's condition still fresh in her mind. After Christmas she returned to her flat in Worthing, which she had taken after selling their house in Totteridge and Bailey's tremendous library of over 4,000 books, with which she had been compelled to part for practically nothing.

On a table at the flat was a stack of Christmas cards. She turned them over with little interest until, at the bottom of the pile she found a letter in Bailey's handwriting.

For years she had received no written communication from Bailey. She tore open the envelope and was astonished at its contents. At the top of the paper was written '24-12-53, 11 a.m.'

Bailey asked her to come and take him out, for he could not understand why he was being detained, having completely recovered. When Veta reached the hospital she was overjoyed to discover that he was quite normal.

The recovery had happened suddenly at 11 a.m. on Christmas Eve. Bailey was not intellectually impaired and the remission was permanent, though for a short period in May 1954 he relapsed into depression with loss of appetite, insomnia and loss of concentration. Apart from this slight temporary setback, he remained normal up to the time of his death.

The doctor in charge of Bailey had also written to Veta enclosing two letters from Bailey, and informing her of his 'remarkable improvement', suggesting a visit and asking her to bring more clothes, but Veta did not receive it.

After Bailey came out of hospital, he and Veta stayed for three weeks at their flat in Worthing and prepared for a trip to the Canary Islands. The preparation consisted mainly of collecting the books and manuscripts necessary for the revision of Bailey's share of the next edition of *Short Practice*. Although Veta feared a relapse they left for Tenerife as soon as they could.

They stayed at Puerta de la Cruz for six weeks, and Veta recalls their puzzlement over the section on irradiation which Bailey was asked (presumably by Mr Love) to write.

'What's this I 131?' he asked Veta. 'Where do I put the 131, before or after the I?' Veta did not know much about it either, but they had brought along all the literature which they could find on irradiation, and after much reading Bailey managed to get the hang of the new nomenclature for radio-active isotopes.

Much new work on them had been done during his illness, but in the end he wrote a short but accurate account of the subject. The whole subject of radio-activity is complicated, but readers unfamiliar with the subject will know that radium is used for treating cancer as its radio-activity kills cancer cells. Iodine, phosphorus, gold, iron, chromium, and cobalt can also be rendered radio-active by disturbing their nuclear arrangement to form isotopes, which are used for diagnosing and treating cancer.

After their 'holiday', Bailey and Veta went back to Worthing where they both continued their share of revision and rewriting of his numerous text books, working, as usual, in separate rooms. But the flat was too small to house all the manuscripts, proofs, illustrations, x-rays, printer's blocks, books and other materials, so they soon moved to a house in Sholden, near Deal, in Kent.

It was part of an enormous mansion, originally St Augustine's Monastery, which had been divided into five separate houses with their own gardens. It was a delightful house, well suited to Bailey's needs, but after four years the Silver City Airways established a route directly over it, close to their landing airfield. The noise of the planes became so intense that Bailey was obliged to stop dictating his manuscripts when a plane passed overhead.

This disturbance compelled them to move again, this time to a bungalow at Alkham, near Folkestone, which was excellent for Bailey as there was a swimming pool and plenty of room in the grounds for him to put up his garden hut. It was also convenient for Veta who by this time was crippled with arthritis and walking with two sticks.

Towards the end of the nineteen-fifties Veta's arthritis was becoming more severe, and Bailey thought that they should get away from some of the worst English winter months. They chose the south of Spain where they bought a plot of land at Fuengirola, near Malaga, and found a builder to build them a house.

Their retreat to Spain was not intended to be permanent, for most of Bailey's work kept him in London, where he spent many hours each day in medical libraries. On their visits to Spain they took with them enough material for continuing the revision of his books.

Throughout his professional life, but especially in his later years, some of Bailey's chief contacts were with librarians, with whom he was popular, although Mr S. Wood, at the Royal College of Surgeons of England, was often harassed by the extra work he provided. In March 1925, while he was at the Liverpool Royal Infirmary, Bailey wrote to Mr Wood, explaining that he had been asked to write a series of articles on surgery in and

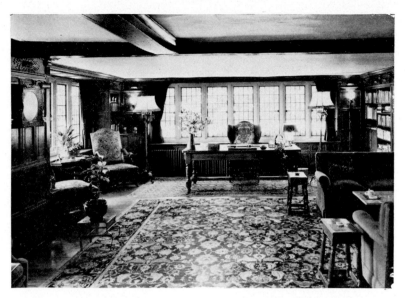

13. The study at Fairlawn, Bailey's second house on Totteridge Common. There were over 4,000 books in this library.

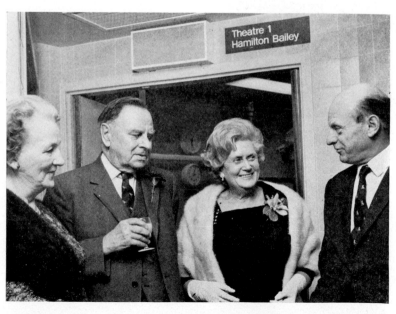

14. The opening of the Hamilton Bailey operating theatre in St David's Wing of the Royal Northern Hospital. Reading left to right: Mrs McNeill Love, Mr R. J. McNeill Love, Mrs Hamilton Bailey, Mr Reginald Murley (Senior Surgeon at the hospital).

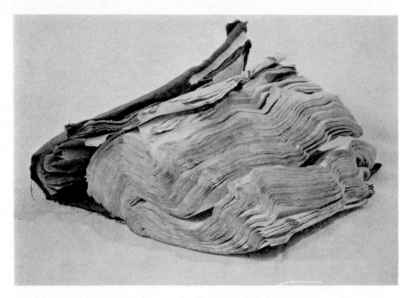

15. A copy of the fifth edition of *Emergency Surgery*, retrieved from the Great Bear Lake by a grateful doctor (see p. 19).

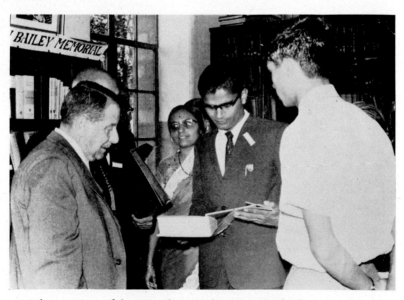

16. The opening of the Hamilton Bailey Memorial Library in Bombay.

around the mouth. He included in his letter a list of 25 subjects for *each* of which he required six *good references*. The specially good articles were to be entered in red ink and those illustrated marked with an asterisk. The references were to be provided on yellow cards. He used cards of different colours to correspond with different hospitals.

Later, Bailey wanted a full reference to suicidal cut throat, a list of books in French and English upon the surgery of the mouth and jaws, and a list of books on surgery for dental students. Afterwards he wrote to Mr Wood again for still more references on a wide variety of subjects. Payment was generous but Mr Wood's difficulty was that he could not find time to do the work.

He remembered Bailey well. He found him demanding in his search for information, yet he seemed to harbour no ill-will, being willing to provide me with all the information which he could about Bailey, and he gave me many letters which Bailey had sent him 45 years before.

The librarians who helped Bailey most with his work were Mr T. John Shields of the B.M.A. and Mr W. J. Bishop of the Royal Society of Medicine.

Mr Shields was able to send Bailey articles before they were listed in the Index Medicus (a monthly index of medical periodicals), and draw his attention to new techniques, etc. Shields indexed most of his books except those published in Bristol. He thinks that Bailey's life can be divided into two parts, the division being caused by the tragic death of his son. Several of his colleagues have given me the same impression. Before the death he was an indefatigable worker and expected others to keep pace.

One of his secretaries said that it was common for them to work until the early hours of the morning and sometimes all through the night. He might be working on three revisions of his books and probably writing a new one at the same time.

After his son's death he tried to do even more work to drown his great sorrow, and could not stand the strain. Shields lost touch with Bailey for the years of his illness. Then, one day, he received a letter stating that Bailey would call to see him at the B.M.A. 'It was quite a different Hamilton Bailey who arrived. He had lost a lot of weight, was hesitant and slow of speech, a sick man convalescing.

'From that day until I retired in 1961 Bailey would write to say that he would be in the library on a certain day, and I would put out literature for him on the subjects named in the letter. He came from Worthing, then from Deal, and later from Spain. His health improved rapidly, and by the end of 1960 he was 95 per cent the old Hamilton Bailey. Hamilton Bailey was a gentleman whom I much admired'.

Mr Bishop, besides helping Bailey as librarian at the Royal Society of Medicine, collaborated with him in writing articles to the journals during the last years of his life on Gram, Leishman, Donovan and Reiter, and earlier with his book entitled *Notable Names in Medicine and Surgery*, which was useful to any one wishing to know the meaning of an eponym attached to an operation, sign, test, organ, tissue, duct, tablet, or anything else in medicine or surgery.

Mr Bishop died before I started writing about Bailey, but one of his successors, as librarian to the Royal Society of Medicine, writes, 'Certainly I knew Mr Bailey, but only in the sense that any young library assistant knows a reader who is likely to come up the stairs, two at a time, demanding half a dozen references before he was in the library. There was nothing bullying in the approach; it was simply that of a very busy man. . . .

'In the nineteen-thirties I recognised Hamilton Bailey's chauffeur just as readily as Bailey himself, because he would send his chauffeur along with a list of references, have the books for a night or two, and then be back for a fresh batch.

'He was the sort of man whom I, as a librarian, like to serve. He told me clearly what he wanted. While he did expect one to do one's best, he was never too busy to say "thank you" for the effort; probably in fact one's best tended to be a little better as a result of attempting something for him.'

11

SPAIN AND HIS DEATH

Their departure to the sun of southern Spain in 1961 did Bailey an unexpected good turn, for it taught him at last the art of relaxation. He did not return to active surgery after leaving the hospital, and was now devoting his whole time to writing. He was no longer subjected to the tensions of the operating theatre, anxiety about patients, the everlasting jangle of the telephone, or the strain of night calls.

He became more good-tempered, placid, and amiable generally. Some of his improvement in temperament may have been the outcome of his long illness, for I have known a severe head injury to produce a similar effect.

A young architect and his wife, Mr and Mrs David, whom I met near Fuengirola, told me of a different Bailey from the one described to me by those who knew him before his illness. They described him as a 'big, kind, gentle and considerate man,' who never made the slightest effort to impress them. They called him 'Hamilton' from the start, in spite of the difference in their ages, for the Davids were still in their twenties.

They once asked him to have a look at their child, Rama, and were reassured when he told them that he thought that there was nothing serious the matter. They said he got on well with children, who instinctively liked him, but the nurses of one of the wards of a hospital near London where babies were treated expressed a contradictory view. The explanation probably is that he was liked by most children old enough to talk to him. With small babies I have yet to meet a doctor able to entice the yellers not to yell.

Mrs David was impressed by Bailey's considerateness towards his wife. Veta had forgone a visit to the hairdresser and set her own hair because she thought it necessary to work on his books. Bailey thanked her for sacrificing her morning for his work, and remarked, 'How nice your hair looks.' Mrs David said she hoped that her husband would talk to her in the same gentle way when they had been married for so many years.

Little did Bailey dream when he went to Spain with Veta that his days of usefulness were nearly over. Though he was no longer a consulting surgeon on the staff of numerous hospitals, his fame as an author was worldwide. It has never ceased to amaze me that he could continue to revise his books so well after his illness even though he never entered the wards or operating theatres of hospitals. He seemed to possess telepathic insight into advancement in surgery. It may have been because his own experience had taught him what could go wrong with surgical cases, and that when other authors described new methods of diagnosis and treatment he could pick out those of special importance.

His seventh edition of *Emergency Surgery*, published in 1958, was in my opinion the best of all. It included an appendix containing practical hints on intravenous fluid therapy, blood transfusion, the latest techniques for the treatment of shock, peritonitis, intra-abdominal injuries, intestinal obstruction, head injuries, pulmonary embolism, amputations, and a host of other subjects.

The illness which terminated his life declared itself insidiously. At first even Bailey could not believe that there was anything serious the matter. For four days his bowels did not act, a thing which had never happened to him before, but he felt well in spite of it. 'If any of my patients came to me with this symptom', exclaimed Bailey, 'I would diagnose intestinal obstruction, which at my age is usually caused by cancer of the bowel.' But three out of four of the cardinal symptoms of intestinal obstruction were absent. He felt no pain, did not vomit, and had no abdominal distention. The only definite symptom of obstruction was absolute constipation for four days.

However, they sent for his G.P., who was unfortunately away from home attending a conference in Madrid. Bailey knew no Spanish, and Veta was a beginner. A locum, who could not speak

English, came. He ordered an enema, which was administered by a practicante, without effect.

The only solution seemed to be to consult somebody who could understand him at a hospital where an operation could be performed if necessary. Bailey therefore went to the nearest English-speaking territory, which was Gibraltar.

He told the doctors there of his suspicion that he might be suffering from an obstruction caused by cancer. They took x-rays of the contour of the bowel after the administration of a *barium meal*, from which they reached a diagnosis of diverticulosis. This is not a serious complaint, consisting as it does of the extrusion of small pouches or sacs from the cavity of the bowel. The condition is quite common in elderly people. They did not give a *barium enema*, by means of which the lower part of the bowel can be depicted with x-rays, which would have provided a better view of the suspected pathology than a barium meal. After a four-day stay in hospital he was discharged, still free from pain.

Bailey could not have believed the optimistic decision of his advisers for his own knowledge of intestinal obstruction, on which he was an authority, would have told him that their opinion was fallacious; but wishful thinking may have made him hope that they were right. He was not left long in doubt, for on the second day after leaving hospital he suffered a severe attack of pain. He again called in his G.P. who had returned from Madrid. He at once called a surgical specialist, who instituted an intravenous drip and gastric suction before transferring him to Malaga.

The surgeon who treated him there was an absolutely first-class man, but by this time Bailey's condition was deteriorating. The surgeon removed a cancerous growth, which restored the function of the bowel. Then the complications started: paralytic ileus, adhesions between the bowel loops, perforation of the bowel, faecal fistula, burst abdomen, and oedema of the lungs.

As each complication developed the surgeon and Bailey discussed together what should be done. Four more operations were performed, but to no avail. Bailey suffered a tremendous amount of pain.

With continued lack of improvement, Bailey realised after some days that he was going to die, but his main concern was about the forthcoming publication of the projected editions of his books on which he had been working before the trouble started, especially *Pye's Surgical Handicraft* and *Short Practice of Surgery*. He was more deeply distressed about his failure to finish his work than his imminent death.

He died on 26 March 1961 at the age of 66 of generalised weakness resulting from the numerous complications. During the whole of his last illness Veta remained constantly with him.

I was working at a hospital in Malawi (then still called Nyasaland) when news of his death reached me. It came as a shock for I had not even heard about his illness. Indeed, only a few weeks before, I had received a letter from him answering a few questions which I had put to him about the instruments (mentioned earlier in this story) which he had been so kind as to send me. I admitted to myself that we all have to die, and Bailey was nearing his three score years and ten, but I felt that I had lost my most useful, though distant, adviser.

Whenever in doubt about how I should treat an acute abdominal emergency (and I treated many) I turned up my *Emergency Surgery*. I feared that in subsequent years the book would no longer be the same. Though further editions have appeared, this book, still the best of its kind, lacks the Bailey touch. Nobody could take Bailey's place in the literature of emergency surgery.

My colleagues in Malawi expressed their dismay when I told them of his death, for they, like me, regarded the 'Ham Bailey' in our library as their unfailing guide when in surgical difficulties.

After his death Veta received letters of sympathy from over 100 of his colleagues. One was from the late W. D. Lovelock Jones, who wrote, 'I cannot refrain from telling you what a patient told me this morning about your dear husband. About 23 years ago Mr Hamilton Bailey removed this patient's thyroid in the Royal Northern Hospital, and she was now, this morning, consulting me for some abdominal condition.

'I happened to mention what a beautiful scar it was on the neck and asked her who did the operation. She said that it was "Sir Hamilton Bailey" of the Royal Northern, and she told me what a wonderful man he was.

'I was so glad to hear this tribute to a very great man, and I felt I had to pass it on to you because I am quite sure such remembrances of him will go on for many years to come. I also thought that the accolade that this lady bestowed upon him was more deserved than she and thousands of other patients will ever realise.'

A memorial comprising his framed photograph and an inscribed brass tablet have been put up at the Parque San Antonio hospital at Malaga, and his photograph is hung in the International College of Surgeons.

Veta established the Hamilton Bailey Trust from the royalties of his books whereby £100 a year is being paid to each of eight medical libraries, £750 a year for a travelling scholarship, and a fund to enable young foreign surgeons to go to England to take a higher surgical qualification. The library fund will be continued in perpetuity to expand the libraries of the medical schools in these countries, most of which are in developing parts of the British Commonwealth. The Hamilton Bailey operating theatre was opened at the Royal Northern Hospital in October 1972 by Mrs Bailey.

Bailey's life was fraught with at least four major crises: the threat to his life in 1914; the loss of his left index finger which was expected by many to end his career as a surgeon in 1924; the death of his son in 1943; and his mental illness from 1948–53.

All surgeons are faced with serious problems and disasters but Bailey met with more than his fair share especially for a man handicapped by an unstable family background and a neglected childhood.

Whatever his faults, he did more for the human race than many others about whom bulky volumes of praise have been written. To date, this is the first book to be written about Hamilton Bailey, whom I believe was one of the greatest surgeons, authors and teachers of surgery of the twentieth century.

GLOSSARY

ADHESIONS: bands holding structures together, especially in the abdominal cavity.

ASPIRATION: suction.

AUSCULTATION: examination with a stethoscope.

AUTOTRANSFUSION: transfusion involving re-introduction of patient's own blood.

BARIUM ENEMA: given to render the lower part of the bowel opaque to x-rays so that abnormalities can be detected.

BARIUM MEAL: barium is swallowed and the digestive tract is x-rayed at intervals to demonstrate the passage of the barium.

BRANCHIAL CYST: found at the side of the neck, of developmental origin.

CALCULI: stones, found in disease of gall bladder, kidney, ureters, urinary bladder, urethra and salivary ducts.

CANNULA: instrument through which fluids can be administered or withdrawn.

CARCINOMA: cancer.

CARDIAC ARREST: cessation of the heart beat.

CARDIAC MASSAGE: rhythmic pressure on the heart to restore its pulsations in cardiac arrest, by either pressure to the chest (external cardiac massage) or by opening the chest (internal cardiac massage).

CAROTID ARTERY: transports blood to the head and neck.

CATHETER: tube for introduction through a narrow canal into a cavity, eg, urethral catheter for evacuating urine from the bladder.

CYSTOSCOPE: instrument ensheathing a telescope through which the bladder can be examined via the urethra and operations performed.

DIATHERMY: use of high frequency current with an electrode for cutting tissues or arresting haemorrhage.

DIVERTICULOSIS: existence of small pouches protruding outwards from within the bowel, liable to become infected, but often harmless.

DRAINAGE TUBE: tube inserted through a wound, usually for providing exit of pus, as after incision of an abscess.

DRIP: medication administered slowly through a tube, usually into a vein, eg, intragastric milk drip, administration of fluid into the stomach.

ECTOPIC PREGNANCY: pregnancy occurring outside the uterus.

ELECTROCARDIOGRAPH: instrument for graphic recording of the heart beat.

ELECTROCOAGULATION: platinum wire heated electrically is passed via a cystoscope into the bladder to destroy tumours.

ELECTRO-CONVULSANT THERAPY (E.C.T.): administration of electric shocks, used in treatment of mental disorders.

EMBOLISM: obstruction of a blood vessel by a blood clot or other substance.

ENDOTRACHEAL ANAESTHESIA: administration of an anaesthetic directly into the trachea (wind-pipe) through a tube.

FAECAL FISTULA: escape of faeces from the bowel externally or into another hollow organ.

FLAVINE: (acriflavine) is a mild antiseptic.

FOMENT: apply fomentations, usually lint soaked in hot water wrung out until almost dry.

GASTRIC SUCTION: a thin rubber or plastic tube is passed through the nose into the stomach, so that contents of the stomach can be sucked out.

GENITO-URINARY ORGANS: organs concerned with reproduction, and excretion of urine.

GRAVES'S DISEASE: (exophthalmic goitre) disease of the thyroid gland, characterised by protrusion of the eyeballs, rapid pulse and loss of weight.

HOMEOPATHIC: branch of medicine which believes in the treatment of some illnesses with drugs in minute doses.

HUNTERIAN PROFESSORSHIP: a surgeon may be made a Hunterian professor of surgery of the Royal College of Surgeons of England for outstanding work.

HYSTERECTOMY: removal of the uterus.

INTERCEPTOR: glass connection with a dropper by which the number of drops of fluid given can be counted.

INTERCOSTAL SPACE: space between two ribs.

INTRAVENOUS SALINE: salt water given into a vein to combat dehydration, which can be caused by excessive sweating, diarrhoea or vomiting.

INTUSSUSCEPTION: portion of the bowel, often quite high up, gets pushed down into the bowel below it, similar to the appearance of a sock with the foot pushed into the leg, ready to put on.

ISOTOPE: chemical element having the same atomic number as the raw element (ie, the same number of nuclear protons) but possessing a different atomic weight (ie, a different number of nuclear neutrons).

I 131: radio-active isotope of iodine with an atomic weight of 131. The atomic weight of iodine is 126.9.

LEUCOTOMY: operation of cutting the front part of the brain.

LIGATURE OF A VESSEL: tying it to prevent bleeding.

LUMBAR PUNCTURE: introduction of a needle into the 'water cushion' surrounding the nerves which extend from the lower part of the spinal cord downwards, eventually to supply the legs and genital organs.

LUMEN: cavity of a tubular structure, eg, the bowel.

MANIC-DEPRESSIVE PSYCHOSIS: characterised by alternating periods of mania and depression.

MESENTERY: layer of tissue suspending the bowel from the back of the abdomen. The mesenteric veins convey blood along the mesentery to the liver.

MASTECTOMY: removal of the breast.

METACARPAL BONE: bone of the hand.

MORPHOLOGICAL: relating to structure.

NEUROMA: tender tumour of nerve tissue.

OEDEMA: swelling or water-logging.

PALMAR SCAR: scar of the palm of the hand.

PARALYTIC ILEUS: condition of extreme distention of part of the bowel, occurring spontaneously, most often after abdominal operations. Cause is obscure.

PAROTIDECTOMY: removal of the parotid gland.

PAROTID GLAND: salivary gland situated in front of and below the ear. It becomes enlarged in mumps.

PATHOLOGY: science of disease or diseased organs and tissues.

PERITONITIS: inflammation of the peritoneum, a membrane lining the inside of the abdominal wall and abdominal organs.

PHALANX: bone of finger. Plural 'phalanges'.

PHYSICAL SIGNS: signs which the surgeon or physician can observe himself without the aid of laboratory tests, x-rays, or other accessory means.

PHYSIOLOGY: science of the functions of the body.

PORTAL SYSTEM: the veins are conduits for blood to pass from most parts of the body straight back to the heart. Blood from the bowel goes first via the portal vein to the liver.

PROSTATECTOMY: removal of the prostate gland which lies at the bladder exit.

PROSTATIC BED: raw surface left after removal of the prostate.

PSYCHOSIS: denotes the more serious behaviour disorders.

PULMONARY: relating to the lungs.

RADICAL OPERATION: aimed at complete cure.

RADIOGRAPHY: the taking of x-rays.

RADIOTHERAPY: treatment with x-rays, radium, or radio-active isotopes.

RELAXANTS: used to prevent muscular contraction during anaesthesia. Helps the surgeon, and the anaesthetist who can more easily pass the endotracheal tube.

REGISTRAR: senior, sometimes resident, doctor in a large hospital.

RENAL VEIN: takes blood to a large vein which in turn goes straight to the heart.

SALINE: fluid consisting of salt dissolved in water.

SCHIZOPHRENIA: mental disease characterised by confusion as to time, place, or identity, and loss of contact with reality.

SPLENIC VEINS: carry blood from the spleen to the liver.

STERNAL PUNCTURE: introduction of a hollow needle or trocar into the bone marrow of the sternum or breast bone to obtain a specimen of bone marrow, or to administer saline or other fluids to the patient when the veins are too small or collapsed.

STREPTOCOCCUS: virulent organism responsible for many diseases.

TALCUM: soft, greasy-feeling magnesium silicate.

THYROIDECTOMY: removal of the thyroid gland in front of neck.

TROCAR: sharp instrument which goes inside a cannula to make a path for it through the tissues.

TUMOUR: a growth, whether benign (comparatively harmless) or malignant (cancerous).

UMBILICUS: navel.

URGENCY ORDER: used when a patient is confined to a mental institution on the request of a relative and the provision of a medical certificate. It remains in force for 7 days.

UROLOGY: surgery dealing with diseases of the urinary organs.

INDEX